THE WORLD'S
FITTEST COOKBOOK

ROSS EDGLEY

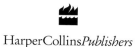
HarperCollins*Publishers*

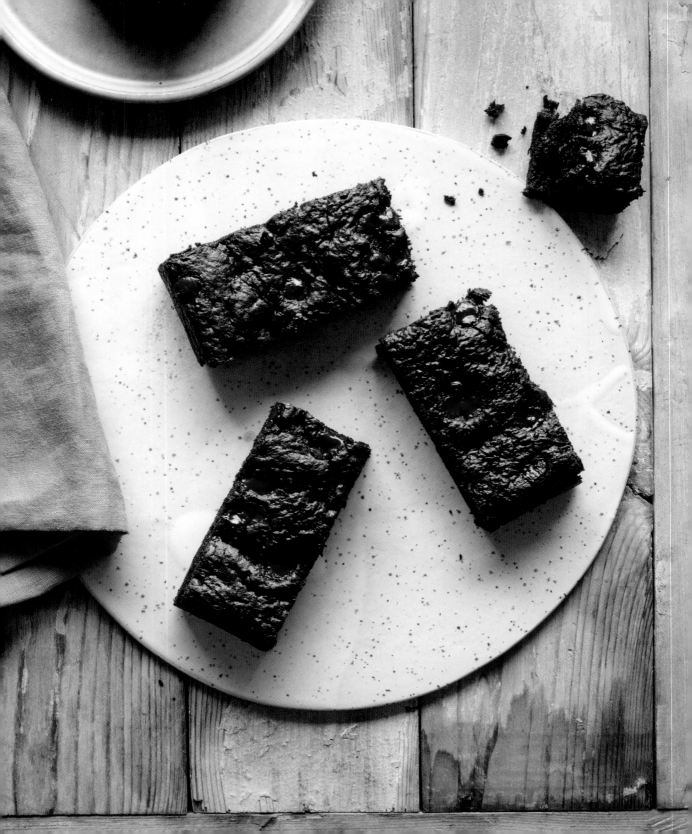

Contents

Introduction

Why 90% of Diets Fail

'Eating is easy.
Nourishment is hard.
Dieting is impossible.'

We've forgotten how to eat.[1]

A bold statement, I know, but in 2018 I broadcast this fact to the world in *The World's Fittest Book* only to have it later (unfortunately) supported by more studies and statistics[2]. As a result, the book became a best-seller, was translated into many languages and I was invited to universities around the globe to talk about how we can fix the failing relationship we have with our fridges.

Essentially, food is not the issue ... our relationship with it is. This is because fat is now feared, calories are confusing and the word sugar has become slander. As a result, unscrupulous personal trainers, celebrities and nutritionists prey on the confused and the desperate. They sell diet plans, promises and 'silver bullet' solutions, despite overwhelming evidence showing they simply don't work[3] and that 90% of diets fail.[4]

There is no single cure or cause for obesity and poor nutritional habits.

Instead, there are many factors at play and each of these is interconnected. This is why the UK Government published an 'obesity map' to illustrate the proverbial minefield that many people find themselves trying to navigate.

'It is now no exaggeration to state that obesity is an international epidemic.'

What's Behind the Obesity Epidemic

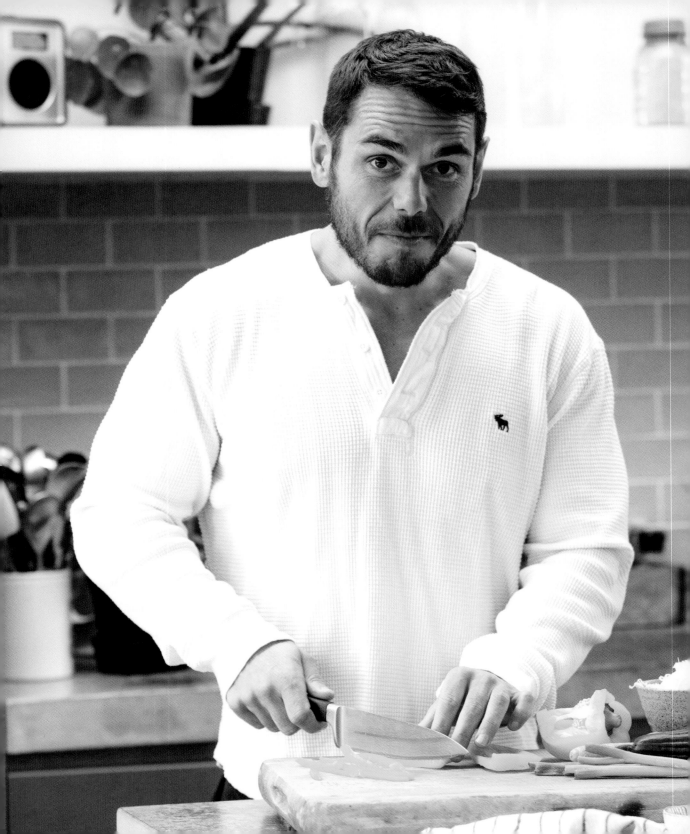

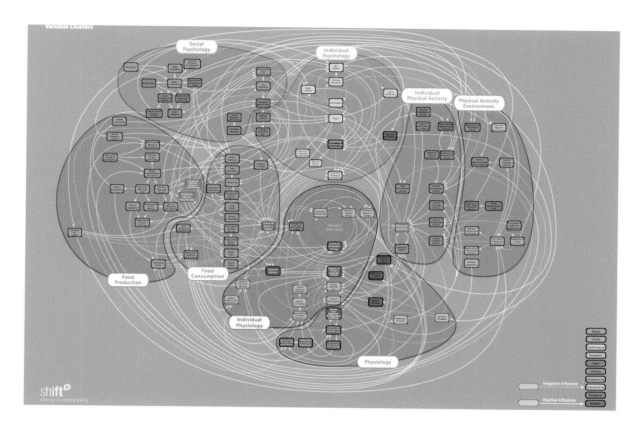

It's a mess, right?

Where *The World's Fittest Book* demystified the core principles of fitness and sports science, *The World's Fittest Cookbook* takes you to the next stage of your health and fitness journey by:

- **Bringing clarity to your food and fridge**
- **Teaching you how to bake, roast and flavour your fat loss**
- **Equipping your kitchen with heaps of incredible nutrient-dense, calorie-controlled recipes**

The goal is to make food only as complicated as it needs to be, not as complicated as it *can* be. This all starts by learning 'The Foodamentals' of fat loss.

The
Foodamentals

THE **NAKED TRUTH**

We are all born naked.

We arrive in this world without any prejudices or preconceived ideas. We don't care about the calorie content of breast milk. Nor do we wonder if there's a 'low-fat' alternative. Equally, we're completely unfazed when the midwife places us on the scales and then announces our weight to the friends and family in attendance.

Yes, life is pretty good!

This is partly because our relationship with food is much simpler. It could be argued that we're actually incredibly in tune with our bodies at this early moment in our lives. Untainted by the latest diet craze, we simply cry to make it known we're hungry and turn our heads when we aren't.

This is why the famous psychologist Abraham Maslow once said, 'All the evidence that we have indicates that it is reasonable to assume in practically every human being, and certainly in almost every newborn baby, that there is an active will toward health.' So where does it go wrong?

Why are so many of us overweight, underweight, hungry, bloated and generally dissatisfied with food?

One possible reason is as we grow older modern society makes it very difficult for us to eat correctly. We're taught:

- **To demonise chocolate, yet the Mayan civilization believed cocoa was sacred.**
- **To monitor our relationship with gravity (weight), when we should really be measuring fat.**
- **To 'battle' cravings, when we should, in fact, be listening to these key biological signals.**

The list goes on, yet studies[5] show if you better organise your fridge you better organise your life.[6]

How do you do this? You must form dietary habits that appease your inner chef, nutritionist and personal trainer. By doing this you ensure you eat according to the laws of:

Gastronomy: studied by chefs, this field of research ensures what you eat tastes good, with flavours, textures and taste all balanced on your plate and palate, so you form dietary habits that you enjoy and can therefore stick to without any effort.

Thermodynamics: studied by personal trainers, this field of research ensures what you eat is calorie-controlled, as any calories (energy) consumed are balanced and considered with calories (energy) burnt through training, so you manage body fat.

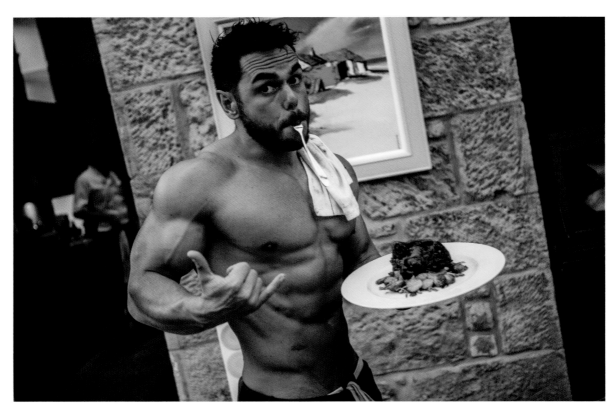

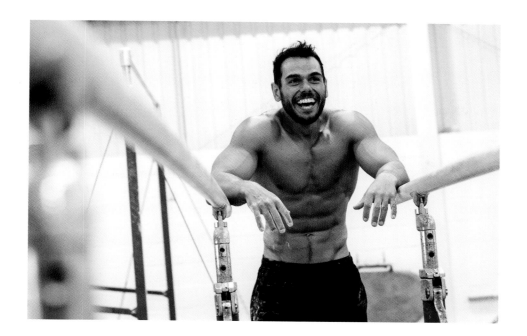

Dietetics: studied by nutritionists, this field of research ensures what you eat is nutrient dense with macronutrients (protein, fats and carbohydrates), micronutrients (vitamins and minerals) and enzymes – all balanced within the diet so you remain healthy.

Therefore the 'sweet spot' of any nutrition plan is one that embodies all three of the above. Basically, where your tummy, taste buds and training all work in perfect harmony.

But a word of warning!

This 'sweet spot' can be hard to achieve. That's because too often chefs are more concerned with taste, nutritionists can be short-sighted when solely studying nutrients, and personal trainers remain fixated with calories in vs calories out. Which is why to achieve balance, we must take a closer look at all three areas and their different schools of thought.

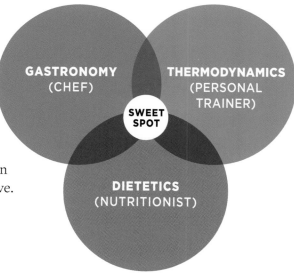

GASTRONOMY (CHEF)

THERMODYNAMICS (PERSONAL TRAINER)

SWEET SPOT

DIETETICS (NUTRITIONIST)

YOUR INNER CHEF
GASTRONOMY

'Enjoyment and taste should not be overlooked or underestimated in any nutrition plan.'

A healthy and happy diet doesn't come from following a rabbit-food diet. Counting and measuring every morsel of food that goes onto your plate is no fun for anyone. Researchers from Louisiana State University found that 'Individuals who engage in rigid dieting strategies reported symptoms of an eating disorder, mood disturbances and excessive concern with body size/shape.' [7]

Put simply, strict dietary habits aren't fun and impact our mental health.

But that's not all, studies rooted in behavioural science also show a boring diet that we don't enjoy eating is doomed to fail. This is based on a large-scale meta study (a study of lots of studies), published by *The International Journal of Obesity,* that concluded, 'Regardless of assigned diet, twelve-month weight change was greater in the most adherent. These results suggest that strategies to increase adherence may deserve more emphasis than the specific macronutrient composition of the weight loss diet itself in supporting successful weight loss.' [8] What this means is when trying to lose fat, the specific diet in question doesn't matter as much, but enjoying it and sticking to it does.

This is why your inner chef is so important. The best diet on paper is useless if you can't follow it in real life. Flavour, taste and texture cannot be ignored. These fundamental truths have a profound impact on the way we eat, yet they are missed by so many nutritionists, who continue to argue whether sweet potatoes are better than white potatoes when in reality this doesn't make a huge difference.

This is why *The World's Fittest Cookbook* has been formulated for big flavour, so you'll want to keep coming back to these irresistible recipes again and again.

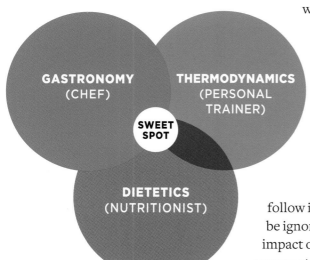

GASTRONOMY (CHEF)

THERMODYNAMICS (PERSONAL TRAINER)

SWEET SPOT

DIETETICS (NUTRITIONIST)

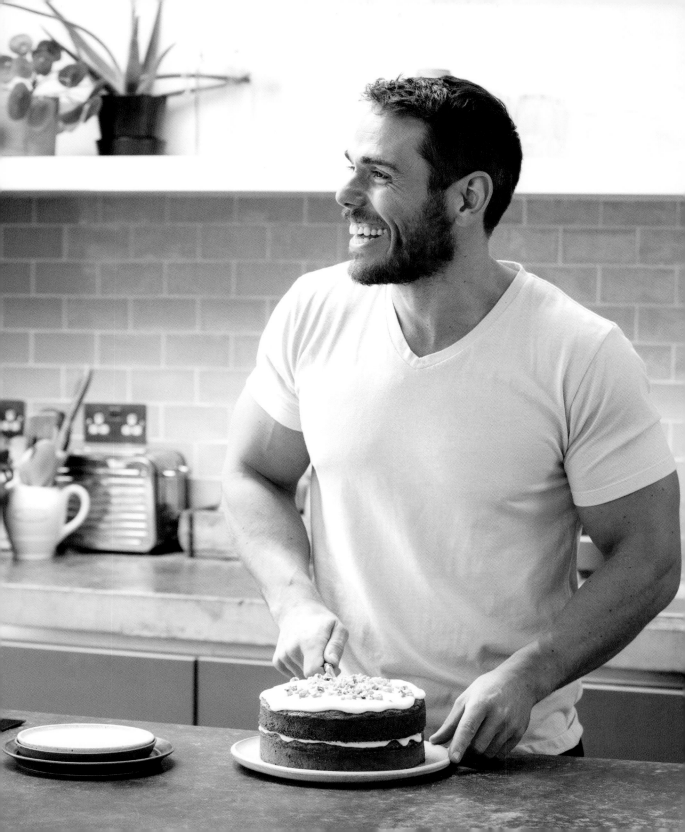

YOUR INNER PERSONAL TRAINER
THERMODYNAMICS

'Don't become emotionally attached to a nutrition or training principle – as sciences progress, so must we.'

Over the years, there have been literally thousands of diets published. Yet, from the many weird and wonderful methods of eating we humans have tasted, tested and trialled, the one thing that all successful diets have in common is they create a calorie deficit (you eat fewer calories than you use).

Whilst many 'experts' might claim their entirely unique approach to eating does something different to achieve fat loss, they are lying. It doesn't. Every single fad and gimmick will only work because in principle you are using more calories (through exercise) than you're eating.

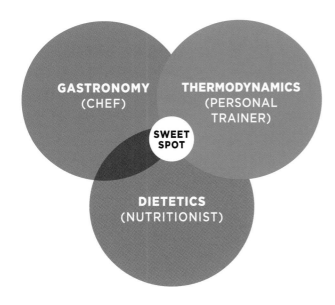

GASTRONOMY (CHEF)

THERMODYNAMICS (PERSONAL TRAINER)

SWEET SPOT

DIETETICS (NUTRITIONIST)

HOW **MAINSTREAM DIETS WORK**

Keto	Consume a diet that's high in fat, moderate in protein and very low in carbohydrates	PUTS YOU IN A CALORIE DEFICIT
Paleo	Consuming organic and naturally occurring foods that our ancestors ate	PUTS YOU IN A CALORIE DEFICIT
Intermittent fasting	Cycle between periods of fasting (complete calorie restriction) and eating	PUTS YOU IN A CALORIE DEFICIT
Low fat	Reducing fat intake	PUTS YOU IN A CALORIE DEFICIT
Weight Watchers	Using a points system and controlled portions	PUTS YOU IN A CALORIE DEFICIT
Sugar free	Avoiding added sugar and reducing naturally occurring sugar	PUTS YOU IN A CALORIE DEFICIT
Whole 30	Focusing on whole foods and avoiding sugar, grains and dairy	PUTS YOU IN A CALORIE DEFICIT
Warrior diet	Eating raw fruit and veg in the day and one big meal in the evening	PUTS YOU IN A CALORIE DEFICIT

The strange thing is we've known about calorie deficits for years. The first ever published definition of the calorie was in a Parisian journal in 1825. This was when Professor Nicolas Clément-Desormes proposed a theory that steam engines converted heat into energy for work. But to validate his theory he needed a unit of heat. Therefore, his first task when calculating fuel efficiency was to define how much energy was contained in fuels.

It was then (when exploring this idea of calorimetry with his head in an engine) that Clément provided the following definition, 'One calorie is the amount of heat needed to elevate by one degree centigrade one kilogram of water.'

Years later, the calorie was being used to quantify the energy content of food.

This is because a pioneer of nutrition called Wilbur Olin Atwater expanded on Nicolas Clément's steam-engine-inspired idea of the calorie. Atwater applied the calorie to nutrition through, 'The systematic chemical analysis of foods'[9] and introduced the concept to the US public in 1887.

Now, our understanding of calories in food has expanded even further. We understand that once we eat food, our body is capable of mainly doing only two things with the calories (energy) from it.

1. You burn it

2. You store it

Understanding this is key to mastering fat loss and fat gain. This is because:

- **If you eat more calories than you burn, you store fat. This is called a calorie surplus.**
- **If you burn more calories than you eat, you lose fat. This is called a calorie deficit.**
- **If you eat the same as you burn, you stay the same. This is called a calorie balance.**

CALORIES IN	CALORIES OUT

Calorie deficit → 2,000 → 2,500 → = Lose weight

Calorie maintenance → 2,000 → 2,000 → = No change

Calorie surplus → 2,500 → 2,000 → = Gain weight

It's that simple.

It's often made to sound more complicated, but research from the Department of Nutritional Sciences at the University of Wisconsin-Madison, USA, states that this is fundamental to fat loss. 'Energy (calorie) balance equation has served as an important tool ... Based on one of the most fundamental properties of thermodynamics it has been invaluable in understanding the interactions of energy intake, energy expenditure, and body (fat) composition'[10].

Losing fat really is just the manipulating of food and fuel within the body. How you do this exactly is entirely up to you.

To prove this, in 2013 I decided to trial three types of diet:

- **High-carbohydrate diet (20% protein, 10% fat and 70% carbohydrates)**
- **High-fat diet (20% protein, 70% fat and 10% carbohydrates)**
- **Balanced macro diet (20% protein, 25% fat and 55% carbohydrates)**

Playing any and every sport I could, my body remained the same at 8% body fat. The only thing that changed was the quantities of the macronutrients I ate. Allow me to show you in a Table of Theoretical Nutritional Awesomeness so you can see a working example of the theory.

NAME: Ross Edgley
AGE: 27 HEIGHT: 5'10 (178cm) WEIGHT: 90kg
TOTAL CALORIES: 3,823 calories per day

HIGH-CARB			BALANCED MACROS			HIGH-FAT		
(Inspired by *The Journal of Sports Medicine*[11])			(Inspired by research from *The Journal of the American Dietetic Association*[12])			(Inspired by *The European Journal of Applied Physiology & Occupational Physiology*[13])		
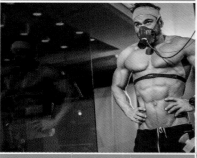			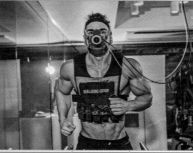			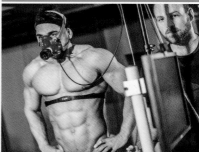		
20% protein	10% fats	70% carbs	20% protein	25% fats	55% carbs	20% protein	70% fats	10% carbs
765 calories of protein	382 calories of fats	2676 calories of carbs	765 calories of protein	956 calories of fats	2103 calories of carbs	765 calories of protein	2676 calories of fats	382 calories of carbs
191g of protein a day	42g of fats a day	669g of carbs a day	191g of protein a day	106g of fats a day	526g of carbs a day	191g of protein a day	297g of fats a day	96g of carbs a day

YOUR INNER NUTRITIONIST
DIETETICS

We twenty-first-century humans are now overfed and undernourished.

If this sounds contradictory, that's because it is. How in the continual harvest that our 'super' markets offer, are we not getting the vitamins, minerals and nutrients our bodies need? To share research published in *The Journal of Obesity Surgery*, 'It is a common belief that clinical vitamin or mineral deficiencies are rare in Western countries because of the unlimited diversity of food supply. However, many people consume food that is either unhealthy or of poor nutritional value that lacks proteins, vitamins, minerals and fibre. The prevalence of vitamin deficiencies in the morbidly obese population is higher and more significant than previously believed'[14].

In a nutshell: we're consuming calorie-dense foods void of nutrients [15].

For this simple reason, we need a new approach to nutrition! Why? *The American Journal of Clinical Nutrition* explains, 'The evolutionary collision of our ancient genome with the nutritional qualities of recently introduced foods may underlie many of the chronic diseases of Western civilisation.'

Our food has changed, but our biology hasn't.

Consider this. Back in the day of our Paleolithic ancestors we were hunters – and to a certain extent foragers and scavengers. Food was in short supply and our survival depended on energy and calories. And thousands of years later, we are still wired to enjoy and seek out foods that are high in fat and sugar. Primitive signals to our brain tell us that this type of food is high in energy and calories and we need it to survive.

But then, we learnt the art of agriculture and animal husbandry – the care, cultivation and breeding of crops and

'Eat nutrient-dense, unprocessed food. Or as our ancestors used to call it, "Food".'

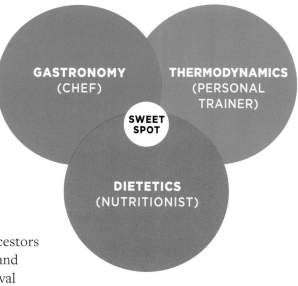

GASTRONOMY (CHEF)

THERMODYNAMICS (PERSONAL TRAINER)

SWEET SPOT

DIETETICS (NUTRITIONIST)

animals. All of a sudden our pantries, and then our fridges, were full of energy and calories. Life was good. Many argue we should have stopped there with our dining tables full of fresh fruit, vegetables and grass-fed cattle. But inevitably we took this all one step further.

We developed, changed and manipulated our food to make it cheaper, to make it faster and to make more of it. Manmade 'food variants' like monosodium glutamate (MSG), trans fatty acids and high-fructose corn syrup were introduced into our diets, despite the human body not recognising them, nor understanding what to do with them.

In fact, many modern forms of tomato sauce, apple juice and ice cream are completely unrecognisable to Mother Nature. She literally has no clue what they are and nor does your body.

Based on this, is it any wonder our bodies are a mess?

Our fridges were once packed full of natural, nutrient-dense foods that have since been replaced with calorie-dense, artificial equivalents. Eating 4,000 calories in a single sitting is now easy with our modern version of food. But I'm willing to bet our caveman ancestors couldn't eat 4,000 calories' worth of shrubbery and fresh meat in one sitting.

This is just the tip of the iceberg. *The American Journal of Clinical Nutrition* adds, 'There is growing awareness that the profound changes in the environment – diet and other lifestyle conditions – that began with the introduction of agriculture occurred too recently on an evolutionary timescale for the human genome to adjust. In conjunction with this discordance between our ancient, genetically determined biology and the nutritional, cultural and activity patterns of contemporary Western populations, many of the so-called diseases of civilisation have emerged. In particular, food staples and food-processing procedures introduced during the Neolithic and Industrial Periods have fundamentally altered crucial nutritional characteristics of ancestral hominin diets.'

For all these reasons and more we need to alter our approach to nutrition, to take into account the environmental and agricultural changes that have occurred in our food.

We must learn to count nutrients as well as count calories.

MACRONUTRIENTS

To do this, we must first gain an understanding of nutrients and how we eat, digest, assimilate and use them within the body. So, what are nutrients? Put simply, a substance used by an organism to survive, grow and reproduce. More specifically, it's macronutrients (protein, fats and carbohydrates), often called 'macros', which we consume in large quantities within the diet that you must develop at least a basic knowledge about.

PROTEIN

THE BASICS

People often associate protein with building muscle. It is, of course, a key part of muscular hypertrophy, but dig a little deeper and you'll find it can help with everything from suppressing hunger to supporting your immune system and overall health.

HOW MUCH DO I NEED?

It's very important to note this is still debated by nutritionists today. The honest answer to this? We don't know. The field of nutrigenomics – how our individual genes uniquely interact with our food – teaches us this varies from person to person. At best, we can make an educated guess and start with research from the often-quoted sports nutrition bible *The Complete Guide to Sports Nutrition*.

It states the International Olympic Committee Consensus on Sports Nutrition recommends strength and speed athletes consume 1.7 grams of protein per kilogram of bodyweight, per day. This is considered the optimal amount to help the muscles repair and re-grow.

CARBOHYDRATES

THE BASICS

Your body gets energy from both fat and carbohydrates. Knowing this is so important because if energy levels are high then losing fat, running marathons and lifting weights all become possible.

But fail to understand it and fat loss becomes hard, impossible or often temporary and you're unable to train with any real intensity as the 'gas tank' is running on empty. So, which one is better? The honest answer is both, since it varies from person to person. But carbohydrates are often referred to as our body's primary fuel source. This is because we're designed to store carbohydrates in the liver, brain and muscles where we can break down the sugar and starch into glucose, which we then use as energy to fuel our bodies and feed our cells.

HOW MUCH DO I NEED?

This depends. Technically, you can live without carbohydrates. But most conventional sports nutritionists would advise against it. This is because we've long known a wholesome bowl of carbohydrate-rich granola in the morning is stored in the muscles as glycogen, ready for us to use later during some form of physical activity.

This idea is supported by the Scandinavian Physiological Society who state, 'Muscle glycogen (carbohydrate availability can affect performance. During both short-term and more prolonged high-intensity intermittent exercise.'[16] And the Australian Institute of Sport agree, writing, 'The recommendations of sports nutritionists are based on plentiful evidence that increased carbohydrate availability enhances endurance and performance during single exercise sessions.'[17]

FATS

THE BASICS

We need fats in our diet to live. Hopefully this is not news to anyone and the low-fat-diet-hype train has well and truly left the station. This is because it's long been shown that our bodies need fat to assist in vitamin absorption, to aid hormone regulation and even aid optimal brain function.

HOW MUCH DO I NEED?

This (again) depends on many factors, but let's look at some research. Firstly, the 2002 report on dietary reference intakes published by The US Food and Nutrition Board (issued jointly by the United States and Canada) quantifies this by stating that healthy dietary fat should constitute 25–35% of calories consumed daily. This would work well as long as there were sufficient carbohydrates in the diet (your other energy-yielding macronutrient).*

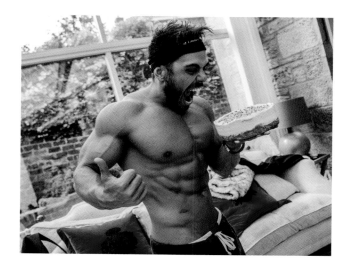

But what about research from *The European Journal of Applied Physiology and Occupational Physiology,* who claim an elite cyclist's performance could be improved by a high-fat diet of 70% fat, 7% carbohydrates and 23% protein, compared to a high-carbohydrate diet of 12% fat, 74% carbohydrates and 24% protein? These results would suggest that two weeks of adaptation to a high-fat diet would result in an enhanced resistance to fatigue and a significant sparing of carbohydrate during low- to moderate-intensity exercise.[18]

What's happening here? Well, the answer is a ketogenic diet (keto).

Low in carbohydrates but high in fat, the goal is to achieve a state of ketosis. This is where the body produces small fuel-efficient molecules called 'ketones' as an alternative fuel for the body when blood sugar (glucose) is in short supply. Basically, they're produced in the liver from fat if you don't have any/many carbohydrates and sugars in the diet and only a moderate amount of protein – since excess protein can also be converted to blood sugar.

The body – and brain – then uses them to fuel the day ahead. Does it work? Again, for some people yes, and for others no. But the theory is fat can become a more efficient fuel source for some people. This is why research published in *Current Sports Medicine Reports* states, 'The number of gruelling events that challenge the limits of human endurance is increasing. Such events are also challenging the limits of current dietary recommendations.'[19] The authors then add that traditionally high-carbohydrate diets have been favoured but there are 'some situations for which alternative dietary options are beneficial.'

HOW TO USE THIS BOOK

Every recipe in this book falls within the 'sweet spot' (with a few exceptions that you'll find and enjoy). This means everything is nutrient-dense, low in calories and tastes amazing – appeasing your inner chef, nutritionist and personal trainer. However, some might be favoured by one more than the others. For instance, the low-calorie, high-protein Chia Seed Peanut Butter & Jelly Protein Pud might appeal just slightly more to your inner personal trainer and nutritionist than your inner chef. While an Oaty Base Banoffee Cheesecake would be welcomed by your inner chef and inner nutritionist, but the (healthy) fat content means the calories would appeal less to your inner personal trainer.

Chia Seed Peanut Butter & Jelly Protein Pud

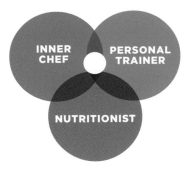

Oaty Base Banoffee Cheesecake

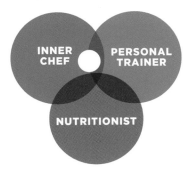

The list goes on, but we encourage you to explore the pages of this book. Think of this book like a buffet, where you can pick and choose from the vast array of options presented to you. Also, don't feel you need to start at the very front … instead, head straight to the recipes that your body needs or your taste buds want. Divided into sections, these include breakfast, lunch, dinner, one-pot wonders, puddings and snacks – so you can create your own tailor-made eating plan.

Finally, within the pages of this book you will find just a handful of recipes that exist outside of the 'sweet spot'. Why? Because my mum is a Jedi grandmaster when it comes to pudding and everyone, once in a while, needs to celebrate a birthday or have a 'blow out' with a calorie-dense dessert. And the only way to do this is with her 'world-famous' cheesecake or rice pudding! Which is why these recipes are included and (unapologetically) only serve to appeal to your inner chef and abide by the laws of gastronomy, and nothing further.

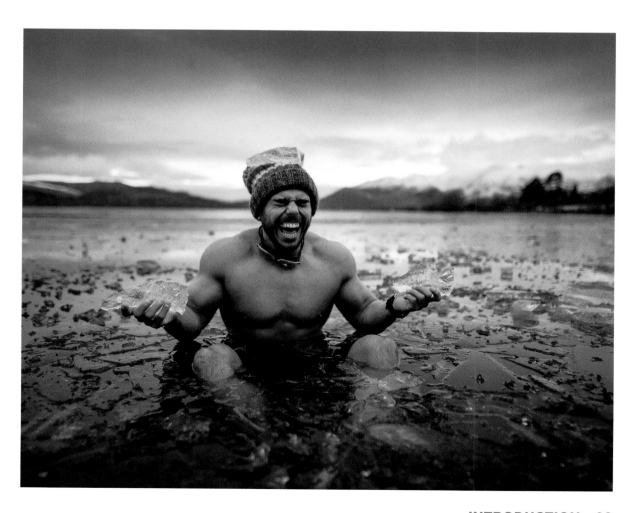

THE EXPERTS

In my 35 years on this earth, it would be hard (almost impossible) to quantify the calories I've consumed throughout my adventures. In fact, it was estimated that in the summer of 2018 I ate over 2 million calories in 157 days to fuel my 1,780-mile swim around Great Britain.

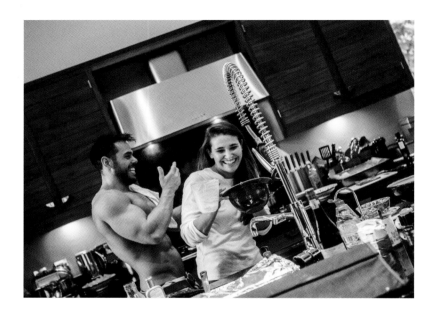

This, combined with the knowledge I gained from four years studying at The Loughborough University School of Sport and Exercise Science and it's clear to see how I've become an (almost accidental) expert in calories, food and fuel.

But despite my academic qualifications and practical application of food and fat loss, I humbly acknowledge my culinary skills pale in comparison to those of Hester Sabery. With First Class Honours in Home Economics & Social Science (essentially food product development combined with an understanding of food behaviour), dove-tailed with additional biomedical science modules, Hester has over a decade of experience working in the food industry. Hester is essentially a black belt in food product development and has created hundreds of recipes for some of Europe's largest food retailers, in which the taste, texture and presentation of food are so important to her. She also happens to be my girlfriend and head chef at home! She taught me to make our famous protein brownies and I now know her recipe by heart.

In contrast, I have worked in sports nutrition for over 15 years, which is why I am mainly concerned with foods and their function. What this means is 90% of the time, if it doesn't help me swim further, lift heavier or recover faster then I'm not interested. Which is why in the nine years we've been together our kitchen has become a battleground. We would argue, debate and fight over whose recipe ideas were the best. But it was the British philosopher Thomas Carlyle who said, 'No pressure, no diamonds', which means when we do agree on a recipe, we create a nutrient-dense, calorie-controlled 'diamond' that tastes incredible. That is how the 'sweet spot' was born. Cross-pollinating ideas from breakfast through to dinner, this book is a giant melting pot designed to accelerate our understanding of food and fat loss.

A NOTE ON INGREDIENTS

The topic of low-calorie sugar replacers continues to divide opinion within the world of dietetics and nutrition. Some people are sceptical of their synthetic nature, whereas others see them as an innovation that can be used to help reduce calories without sacrificing taste. Which is why you'll notice that some of recipes in the dessert section contain them and others don't, so whatever your opinion there will be a collection of sweet solutions to suit your goals.

You'll find there are lots of different types available. We've stated in the recipe whether to use white sugar or brown sugar replacer. We usually use stevia since we like the taste and it's naturally derived from the leaves of the plant species *stevia rebaudiana*. But there are other kinds available (such as erythritol, which is also available in a powdered form to use as an icing sugar) and we'd encourage you to research and experiment with your own form of edible exploration to see what works for your own taste buds and tummy. Some of the recipes also use low-sugar syrups and spreads – the flavours of Sweet Freedom or The Skinny Food Co, which are widely available, are great.

Protein powder is such a great way to make sure your body is getting the protein it needs – not just in shakes but in baking too. We love the flavour of PhD protein powders and usually use whey powder, but plant-based protein powder can also be used in any recipe in this book.

Breakfast

Every breakfast in this section has been taste trialled and battle tested throughout two decades of athletic adventures. From the nutrient-dense, immune-boosting smoothies to the recovery-enhancing, protein-enriched waffles and pancakes, each represents a strong way to start your day.

CALORIES 463
PROTEIN 39g
FAT 12g
CARBS 45g
SUGARS 13g

SERVES
1

Preparation time: 5 minutes
Cooking time: 15 minutes

150g baked beans with no
 added sugar
1 tsp BBQ sauce
½ tsp Worcestershire sauce
½ tsp smoked paprika
2 smoked bacon medallions
80g baby plum tomatoes,
 halved
handful of spinach leaves (25g)
1 egg
1 crumpet
25g 50% reduced-fat Cheddar
 cheese, grated
sea salt and freshly ground
 black pepper
spray light oil for cooking

FULL ENGLISH CRUMPET MELT

A full English with a bit of all your favourites that doesn't take up the majority of your macros for the day! This breakfast/brunch has a fluffy crumpet base, stacked with melted cheese, smoked bacon, smoky beans, sizzled plum tomatoes and spinach, and topped off with a dippy poached egg. Basically, you will struggle to find a crumpet that's packed with as much flavour and protein as this one.

1. In a small saucepan mix the baked beans, BBQ sauce, Worcestershire sauce and smoked paprika, along with a pinch each of salt and pepper. Set over a low heat to warm up while you prepare the rest of the ingredients.

2. Heat a frying pan over a medium heat, spray the base with spray light oil and cook the bacon medallions for a few minutes on each side until cooked through. (Cook for a little longer if you like your bacon crispy.)

3. While the bacon is cooking, add the halved tomatoes to the same pan and fry until they are just starting to catch and are softening up slightly. Add the spinach leaves for the last few minutes of cooking so they wilt slightly.

4. Meanwhile, poach the egg in a saucepan of boiling water for 3–4 minutes until the white is just set.

5. Lightly toast your crumpet, place on a plate and sprinkle the grated cheese on top. Place the bacon on top of the cheese.

6. Pour the beans on top of the bacon and crumpet along with the fried tomatoes and spinach. Add the poached egg and tuck in!

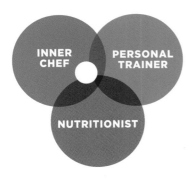

INNER CHEF

PERSONAL TRAINER

NUTRITIONIST

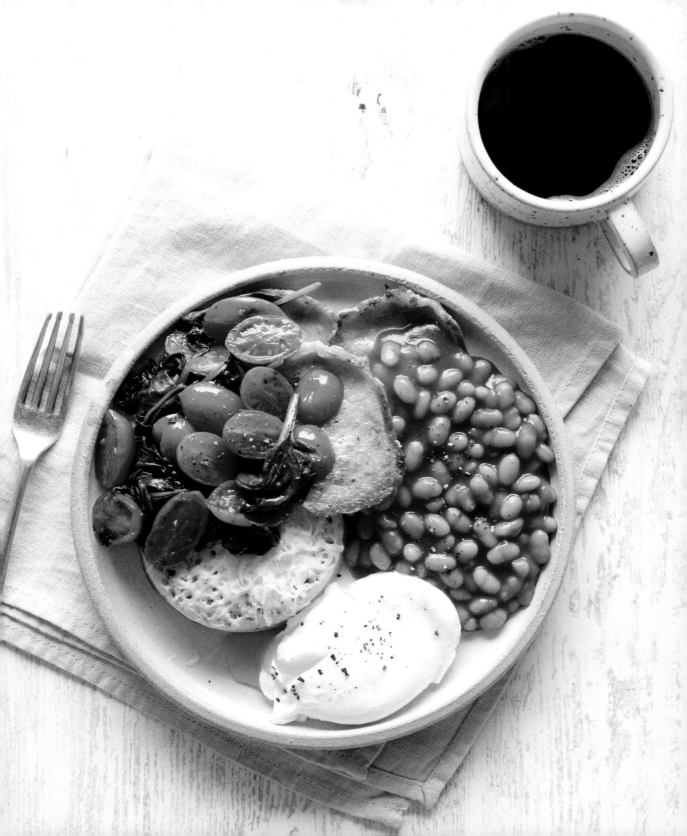

SERVES 1

BLUEBERRY & BANANA OAT BAKE

Preparation time: 5 minutes
Cooking time: 15 minutes

40g rolled oats
1 tsp baking powder
1 tsp ground cinnamon
1 small banana, chopped
50ml almond milk
20g blueberries
2 tsp low-calorie caramel syrup
0%-fat Greek yogurt (optional)
spray light oil for greasing

When I'm in a hurry (or just impatient and getting 'hangry') this is my go-to snacky breakfast. Quick and simple to make, this Blueberry and Banana Oat Bake is a mix between an oaty flapjack and a cake. It has a crispy crust on the outside and a warm, moist centre on the inside that satisfies even the sweetest tooth and keeps you feeling fuller for longer.

1. Preheat the oven to 180°C/160°C fan/gas 4.

2. Combine the oats, baking powder and cinnamon in a bowl and set aside.

3. Mash three-quarters of the banana in another bowl and whisk in the almond milk.

4. Mix the dry ingredients into the banana mixture and stir through a few of the blueberries.

5. Use spray light oil to grease the inside of a mini loaf cake tin and spoon in the mixture.

6. Decorate the top of the oat bake with the remainder of the blueberries and the remaining chopped banana. Place in the preheated oven and bake for 15 minutes until cooked through, golden on top and springy to touch.

7. Remove from the oven and leave to cool in the tin for 10 minutes before serving.

8. Drizzle with the caramel syrup for some extra sweetness and add a dollop of 0%-fat Greek yogurt, if you like.

Tip: If you don't have mini loaf tins you can use a muffin tray. Simply line two of the compartments and split the mixture between them.

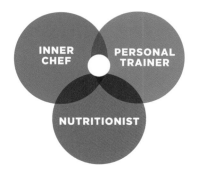

INNER CHEF
PERSONAL TRAINER
NUTRITIONIST

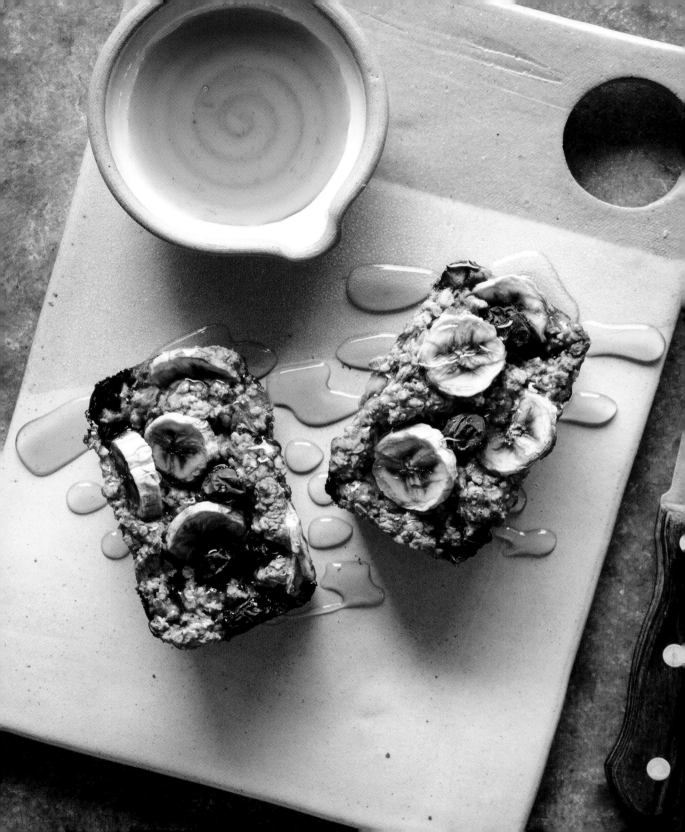

CALORIES 212
PROTEIN 3g
FAT 1g
CARBS 46g
SUGARS 33g

HULK SMOOTHIE

Preparation time: 5 minutes

250g fresh mango, peeled
 and diced (or frozen mango
 pieces)
50g spinach
50g kale
200g fresh pineapple, peeled
 and diced
1 green apple, diced
450ml coconut water
200g ice cubes

It's widely known that athletes have elevated nutritional requirements. And while many people place a focus on calories, protein and macro nutrients, it is equally important to meet your elevated requirements for vitamins, minerals, micronutrients, enzymes and electrolytes. This is exactly why we created this smoothie – it's packed with all the above, making sure your inner nutritionist is happy!

1. Place all the ingredients in a blender and blitz for a minute or so until smooth and creamy.

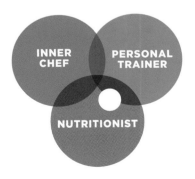

INNER
CHEF

PERSONAL
TRAINER

NUTRITIONIST

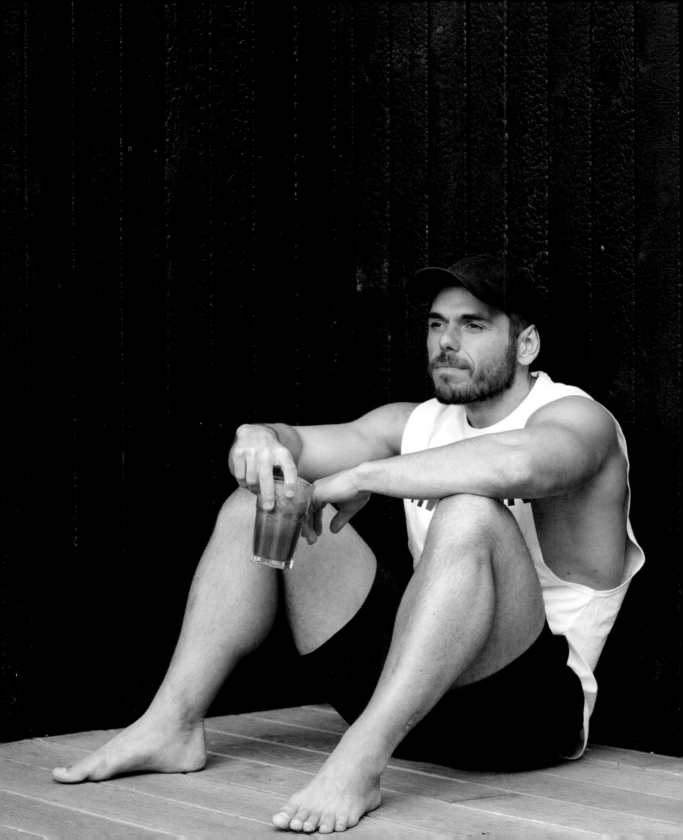

CALORIES 219
PROTEIN 20g
FAT 5g
CARBS 22g
SUGARS 7g

SERVES 2

COFFEE & COCOA PROTEIN MILKSHAKE

Preparation time: 5 minutes + cooling

1 ripe banana
200ml unsweetened oat milk
2 scoops (50g) plant-based chocolate protein powder
1 tbsp cocoa powder
1 tbsp instant coffee granules, mixed with 300ml boiling water and left to cool
2 handfuls of ice

This has to be the simplest and quickest recipe in the whole cookbook! Simply blitz all the ingredients together and then sip or 'skull' it. High in protein, this shake is also a good source of caffeine for anyone needing a pick-me-up before a workout or throughout the day.

1. Place all the ingredients into a blender and blitz until smooth.

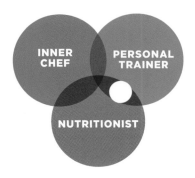

INNER CHEF

PERSONAL TRAINER

NUTRITIONIST

CALORIES 328
PROTEIN 24g
FAT 13g
CARBS 28g
SUGARS 20g

LUSH PROTEIN FROZEN SMOOTHIE BOWL

SERVES 2

Preparation time: 10 minutes

1 small banana, frozen
100ml almond milk
100g frozen raspberries
100g frozen blueberries
2 scoops (50g) vanilla protein
    powder

FOR THE TOPPING
30g dark chocolate
50g smooth peanut butter
25g frozen blueberries
25g frozen raspberries

Sometimes the best way to start the day is to 'flood' the body with nutrients through a frozen smoothie bowl that's densely packed with fruit and protein. Loaded with antioxidants, vitamins and minerals, then enhanced with easily digested whey protein, it's also brilliantly complimented with chunks of rich dark chocolate to cut through the sweetness.

1. Place all the smoothie ingredients in a blender and blitz until it has a smooth, ice-cream-like consistency. Don't blitz for more than you have to, as the more you blitz, the more air is incorporated, which lightens the colour of your smoothie mix. You may find you need to scrape the sides down a few times or give the blender a little jiggle.

2. Place the chocolate and peanut butter in a heatproof bowl over a pan of simmering water, making sure it doesn't touch the water. Gently melt the chocolate and peanut butter, stirring occasionally. (Alternatively, place the bowl in a microwave and heat for no more than 6 seconds at a time, stirring each time until the chocolate and peanut butter has fully melted, taking care not to burn it.) Pour the frozen smoothie mix into your breakfast bowl and scatter the frozen blueberries and raspberries on top before drizzling over the melted chocolate and peanut butter.

Tip: When freezing bananas, slice them and freeze them for a few hours on a flat tray then transfer to an airtight container or freezer bag. This stops the slices from sticking together, making them easier to blitz.

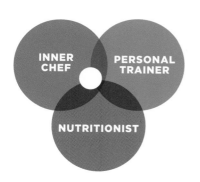

INNER CHEF

PERSONAL TRAINER

NUTRITIONIST

CALORIES 399
PROTEIN 24g
FAT 22g
CARBS 16g
SUGARS 10g

CHIA SEED PEANUT BUTTER & JELLY PROTEIN PUD

SERVES 2

This recipe is AMAZING, since it plays with the boundaries of breakfast and dessert. The fruity tartness of the raspberry jelly combined with the sweet, vanilla peanut butter chia base is naturally high in protein, good fats and antioxidants.

Preparation time: 10 minutes
  plus chilling
Setting time: overnight

300ml almond milk
1½ tbsp (45g) smooth peanut
  butter
1 scoop (25g) vanilla protein
  powder
50g chia seeds

FOR THE JELLY
300g frozen raspberries

TO DECORATE
2 tsp smooth peanut butter
handful of frozen raspberries

1. First make the raspberry jelly. Heat a small saucepan over a low heat, add the frozen raspberries and stir until the raspberries have broken down and are starting to simmer. Immediately turn off the heat and reserve 2 tablespoons of the raspberry sauce for decoration. Pour the remaining fruit sauce into two breakfast pots or ramekins and place in the fridge to cool completely.

2. Mix the almond milk, peanut butter, protein powder and chia seeds together in a large bowl until fully combined, making sure there are no lumps. Gently spoon the chia pudding mix on top of the chilled raspberry jelly bases. Place the chia pots in the fridge overnight to set.

3. In the morning, add a little peanut butter to the top of each of the chia puds and top with the reserved raspberry jelly. Add a few raspberries on top to finish.

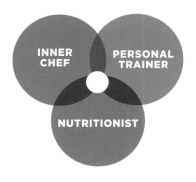

INNER CHEF
PERSONAL TRAINER
NUTRITIONIST

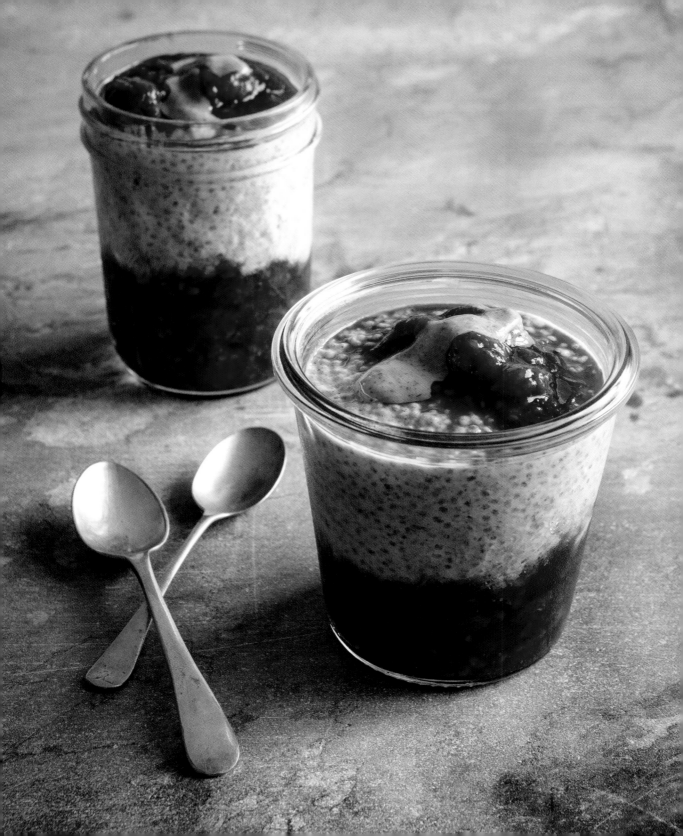

CALORIES 325
PROTEIN 23g
FAT 10g
CARBS 90g
SUGARS 10g

SERVES 2

Preparation time: 5 minutes
Cooking time: 12 minutes

200ml almond milk
1 egg
1 scoop (25g) salted caramel
    protein powder (or any
    flavour you prefer)
1 tsp vanilla extract
1 tsp ground cinnamon
4 slices medium-sliced
    wholemeal bread
80g fresh mixed berries
1 tsp low-calorie chocolate
    syrup
spray light oil for cooking

PROTEIN FRENCH TOAST

The only thing better than French toast is protein-enriched, fruit-infused, cinnamon-dusted French toast! This recipe can only be described as powerful, since it packs a massive 23g of protein into each serving. The best thing about French toast is, of course, the mixed berries soaking into the already sweet and golden wholemeal slices!

1. Whisk the almond milk, egg, protein powder, vanilla extract and cinnamon in a wide mixing bowl.

2. Dip each slice of the wholemeal bread in the mix, making sure you completely coat both sides in the eggy mixture.

3. Place a large frying pan over a medium heat and coat the base with spray light oil. Fry each slice of bread for around 3 minutes on each side until golden and crispy. (You may need to do this in batches if your pan isn't big enough for all four slices at once.)

4. Scatter the berries over your French toast and drizzle with the chocolate syrup to serve.

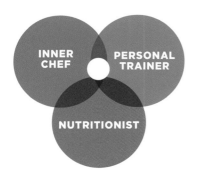

INNER CHEF
PERSONAL TRAINER
NUTRITIONIST

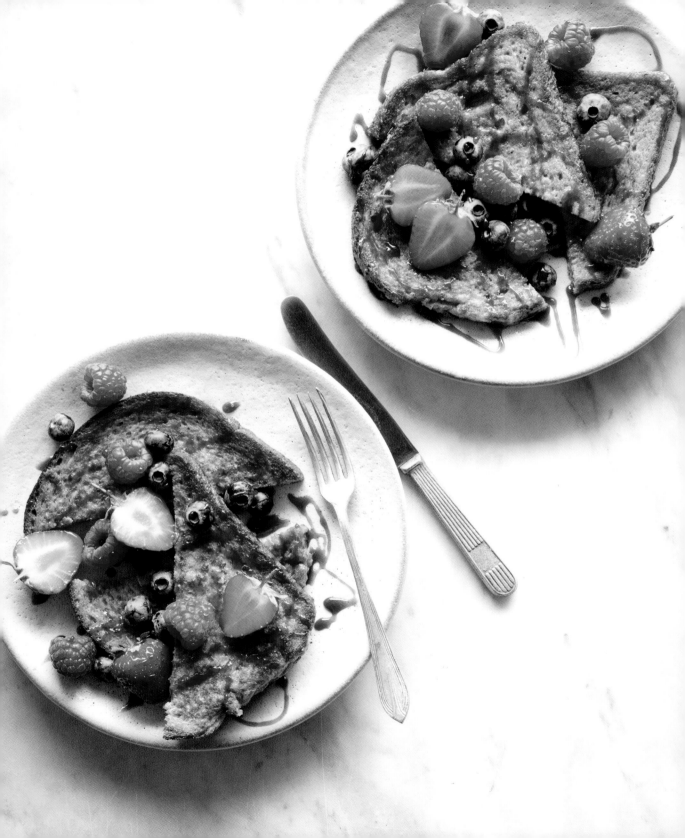

CALORIES 238
PROTEIN 24g
FAT 9g
CARBS 32g
SUGARS 4g

SERVES 2

CLOUD 9 PROTEIN PANCAKES

Preparation time: 10 minutes
Cooking time: 25 minutes

1 egg white
80g self-raising flour
2 tbsp zero-calorie granulated
    white sugar replacer
1 heaped scoop (30g) vanilla
    protein powder
5 tsp (25g) matcha powder
½ tsp baking powder
1 egg
1 tsp vanilla extract
½ tbsp rapeseed oil
180ml soya milk
spray light oil for cooking

FOR THE MARSHMALLOW FLUFF
    (OPTIONAL)
25g powdered gelatine
58ml cold water
1 tsp vanilla extract
185ml boiling water
4 tsp zero-calorie granulated
    white sugar replacer

FOR THE RASPBERRY COULIS
100g frozen raspberries
½ tbsp zero-calorie granulated
    white sugar replacer

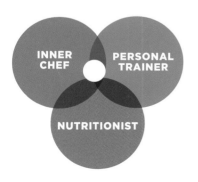

Picking a favourite recipe from this book is impossible, it's like choosing your favourite child. But with that said, Japanese-style matcha cloud pancakes would be your kid who always wins at every school sports day. That's because everything about this breakfast (or brunch) is EPIC! High in protein, served with sugar-free, low-calorie marshmallow 'fluff' and topped with a sweet and sharp raspberry coulis – a breakfast game doesn't come much stronger than this. See photo on the next page.

1. Start by making the raspberry coulis. In a small saucepan, heat the raspberries and sweetener over a medium heat until the raspberries start to break down and the sweetener dissolves. Set the coulis aside until you're ready to serve your pancakes.

2. To make the marshmallow fluff, place the powdered gelatine in a small bowl with cold water to soften and dissolve. In a saucepan, boil the water and mix in the white sugar replacer. Stir until dissolved and then remove from the heat. Give the gelatine a whisk to ensure it is broken up, then add the dissolved sweetener water and vanilla extract. Whisk the mixture until it is thick and fluffy.

3. Heat a non-stick frying pan on the lowest heat possible and coat the base with spray light oil. Keep the pan lid to one side.

4. Using a hand-held electric mixer, whisk the one egg white in a clean mixing bowl until it becomes glossy and stiff peaks form, then set aside.

5. In a separate mixing bowl, beat together the flour, sweetener, protein powder, matcha powder, baking powder, the whole egg, vanilla extract and rapeseed oil. Finally, slowly add the soya milk, mixing in a bit at a time.

6. Use a silicone spatula to gently fold the whipped egg white into the batter mix, taking care not to knock the air bubbles out of the mixture.

7. Place four crumpet rings onto the warmed frying pan and spray the inside of the rings with spray light oil.

8. Pour the pancake mix into the crumpet rings so they are three-quarters full. Place the lid on the frying pan and gently heat for 12–15 minutes. (It's very important that your hob is on the lowest heat possible.)

9. Check the top of the pancakes after they have been cooking for 12 minutes – small bubbles should appear on the surface of the pancake and most of the surface should have dried out slightly. If the surface still looks very moist and uncooked, leave it to cook for a few more minutes.

10. Carefully flip the crumpet ring over so the pancake can cook for a further 2–3 minutes on the other side. Both sides of the pancake should be a lovely golden brown colour.

11. The pancakes should slip out of the crumpet rings with ease, but if they need a little help run a small knife around the edges of the inside of the crumpet ring. Stack your cloud pancakes up on a serving plate and serve with a big spoonful of marshmallow fluff and some raspberry coulis to finish.

Tips: If you don't have any crumpet rings you could use four metal cookie cutters around 8–9cm in diameter. Cooking these pancakes over a very low heat is what helps give them a really lovely light and airy texture. This being said, the lowest heat on different hobs can vary quite a lot, so if your pancakes are taking much longer to cook you may want to increase the heat ever so slightly.

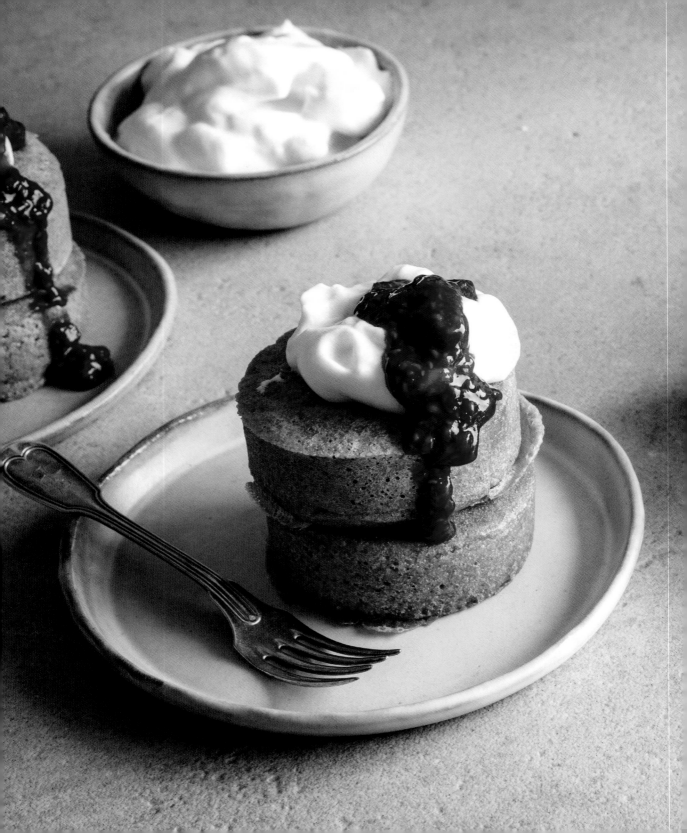

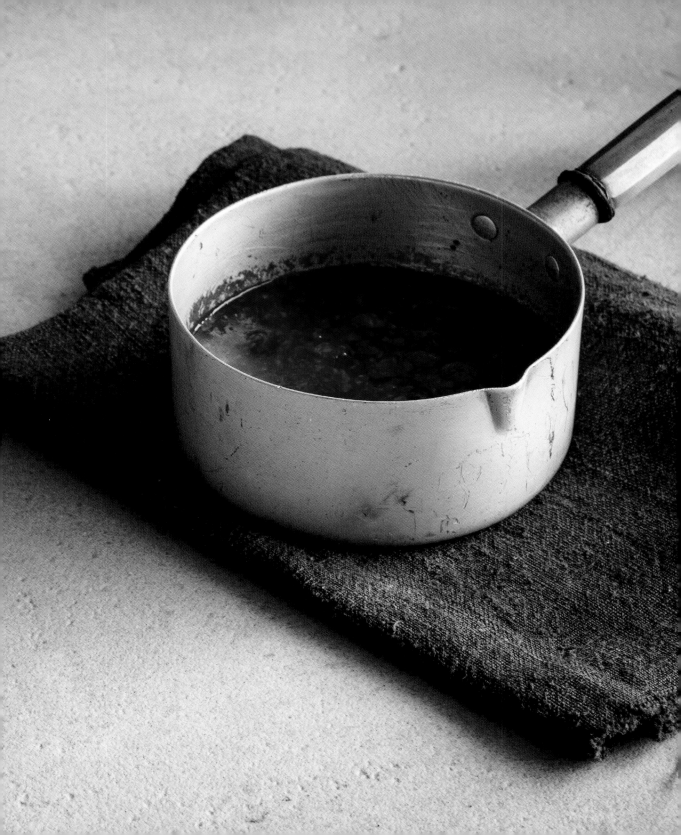

CALORIES 397
PROTEIN 28g
FAT 12g
CARBS 46g
SUGARS 11g

SERVES
1

CHICKEN CHIPOLATA, AVOCADO & CARAMELISED ONION BREAKFAST BURGERS

Preparation time: 15 minutes
Cooking time: 20 minutes

50g avocado
1 red onion, thinly sliced
2 tbsp balsamic vinegar
1 tsp zero-calorie granulated white sugar replacer
3 low-fat chicken chipolata sausages
1 English muffin
sea salt and freshly ground black pepper
spray light oil for cooking

I love burgers. In fact, I love burgers so much I have them for breakfast and this particular one is my favourite. Sweet and salty, it's a strong start to the day, delivers 28g of protein per serving and is a solid source of carbohydrates and healthy fats. I remember when Hester first made us these on a Sunday morning, she walked away from them for just a few seconds and came back to crumbs! Both of them!

1. In a small bowl, mash the avocado, season with a little salt and pepper and set aside.

2. Lightly coat the base of a small frying pan with spray light oil and on a medium heat fry off the red onions until softened. Add the balsamic vinegar and sweetener and let the onions simmer for a further few minutes, stirring to ensure all the onions are enrobed in the sweet vinegar mixture. After a few minutes the onions should be a lovely dark caramelised colour with a sticky textured sauce. Turn off the heat and set aside.

3. Squeeze the meat out of the sausage skins and mould it into a burger patty. Spray a little spray light oil into a frying pan and set over a medium heat. Fry the patty for 3–4 minutes on each side until cooked through.

4. Halve and toast the muffin. Spread the avocado on the bottom of the muffin, place the chicken burger on top then spoon over the balsamic onions. Top with the remaining half of the muffin and enjoy warm.

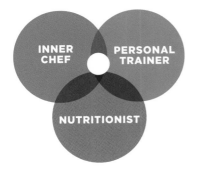

INNER CHEF
PERSONAL TRAINER
NUTRITIONIST

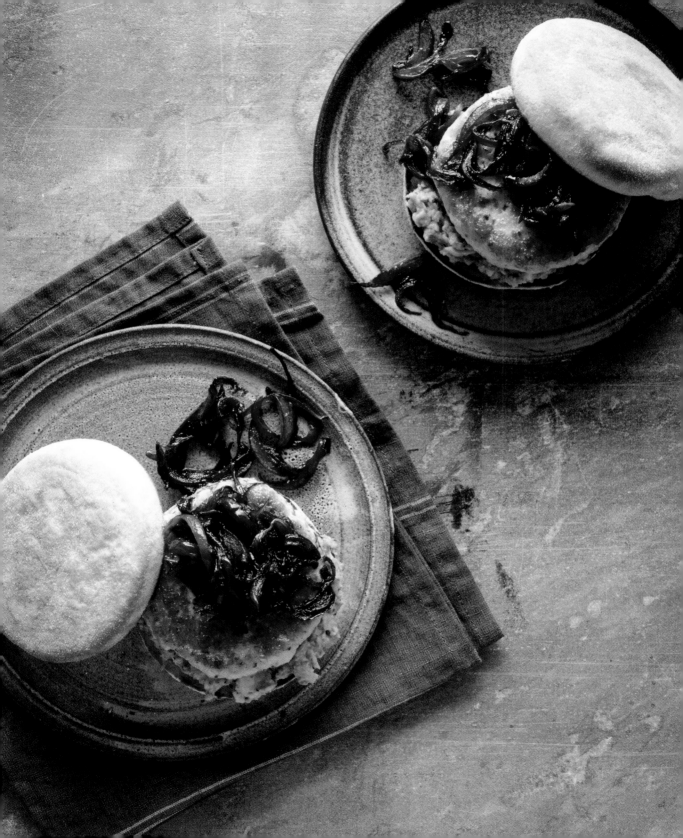

CALORIES 357
PROTEIN 31g
FAT 7g
CARBS 35g
SUGARS 11g

BANANA PROTEIN SCOTCH PANCAKES

SERVES 2

Preparation time: 5 minutes
Cooking time: 12 minutes

100ml almond milk
60g self-raising flour
60g banana-flavoured protein powder
1 tsp baking powder
1 egg
spray light oil for cooking

TOPPINGS
1 small banana, sliced
2 tsp low-calorie flavoured syrup of your choice

Scotch protein pancakes are so versatile and can be topped and decorated with just about anything. We normally go for a form of low-calorie sweet syrup drizzle, or (equally as tasty) add a nut butter spread if you want to include some healthy fats in your diet.

1. Using a balloon whisk, beat all the pancake ingredients together in a large mixing bowl to make a thick and smooth batter.

2. Heat a non-stick frying pan over a medium heat and lightly coat the base with spray light oil.

3. Spoon a small ladleful of batter into the frying pan and cook for 2–3 minutes on each side until golden brown. You should be able to tell when the first side is cooked as little bubbles will start to form on top of the batter. Repeat until all the batter is used.

4. Decorate your pancakes with slices of banana and a drizzle of low-calorie flavoured syrup (we like caramel or popcorn flavoured, but anything goes!).

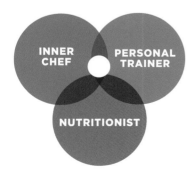

INNER CHEF
PERSONAL TRAINER
NUTRITIONIST

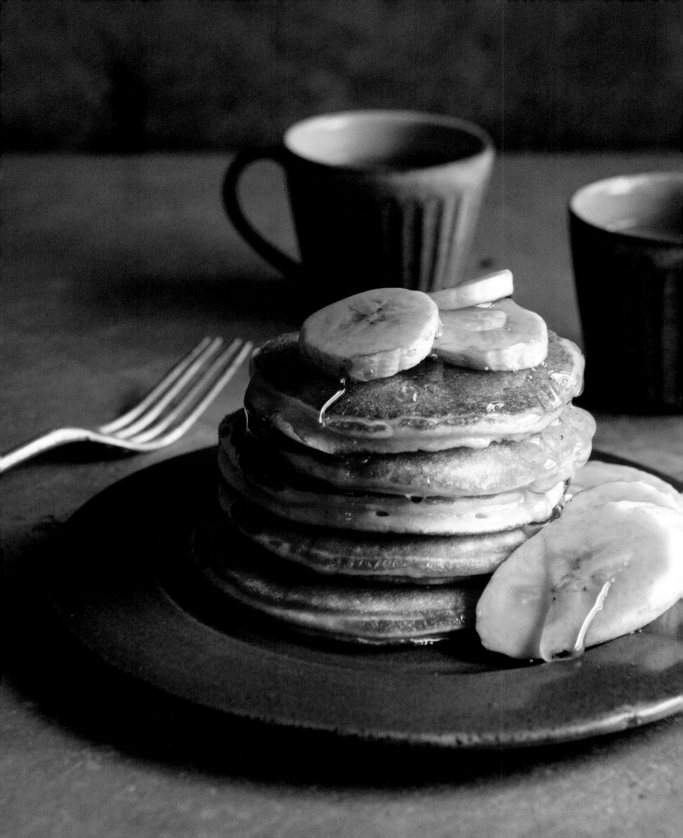

CALORIES 207
PROTEIN 8g
FAT 5g
CARBS 31g
SUGARS 10g

HIGH-FIBRE HIDDEN-CENTRE PROTEIN BREAKFAST MUFFINS

MAKES 12

Preparation time: 10 minutes
Cooking time: 25 minutes

300g butternut squash, peeled and chopped
60g apple sauce
50g maple syrup
3 eggs
60g pumpkin seeds
40g rolled oats
260g wholewheat self-raising flour
20g ground flaxseed
2 tsp bicarbonate of soda
2 tsp baking powder
1 scoop (25g) vanilla protein powder
1 tsp ground ginger
2 tsp ground cinnamon
50g grated apple
60g blackcurrant jam

This wholesome butternut squash and apple breakfast muffin will be your secret weapon when combatting cravings (and it goes perfectly with a freshly brewed cup of tea). High in fibre and a great source of protein, the fruity jam hidden centre serves to satisfy your sweet tooth.

1. Preheat the oven to 180°C/160°C fan/gas 4 and line a 12-hole muffin tin with muffin cases.

2. Place the butternut squash in a bowl and microwave on high for 4–5 minutes until soft. Mash the squash until smooth then set aside to cool a little.

3. Using a hand-held electric mixer or stand mixer, beat together the mashed butternut squash, apple sauce, maple syrup and eggs.

4. Set aside half the pumpkin seeds and 1 tablespoon of rolled oats for sprinkling on top of the muffins then add the remaining pumpkin seeds and oats to the rest of the dry ingredients and mix together with a fork.

5. Pour the mixed dry ingredients into the butternut squash mix and stir together. Finally, stir in the grated apple.

6. Split the batter between the 12 muffin cases then sprinkle the reserved rolled oats and pumpkin seeds on top. Place the muffins in the oven for 25 minutes until they are golden brown and springy to touch.

7. Remove from the oven and leave the muffins to cool in the muffin tray.

8. When the muffins are completely cool, take the papers off. Add the jam to a piping bag, place into the base (you may need to make a little hole first with the end of a teaspoon) and squeeze into the muffins' bases to create a hidden centre. Alternatively, use a small serrated knife to slice off a small section of the top of the muffin, spoon a teaspoon of jam onto each muffin then gently place the muffin lid back on.

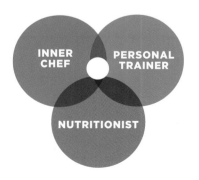

INNER CHEF

PERSONAL TRAINER

NUTRITIONIST

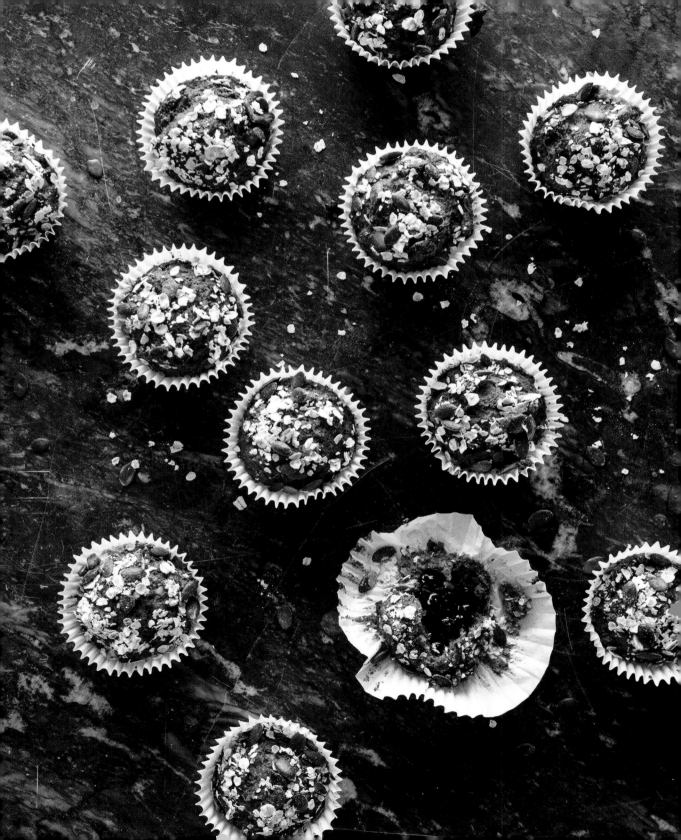

CALORIES 207
PROTEIN 8g
FAT 5g
CARBS 31g
SUGARS 10g

SERVES 1

Preparation time: 10 minutes
Cooking time: 10 minutes

1 tbsp green pesto
1 wholemeal tortilla wrap
½ red onion, finely chopped
30g baby plum tomatoes,
  halved
150g (about 5) egg whites
handful of baby leaf spinach
  (25g)
15g feta cheese
15g mature Cheddar cheese,
  grated
1 tbsp Flora Light spread
  (or other light spread)
sea salt and freshly ground
  black pepper
spray light oil for cooking

CHEESY EGG WHITE BREAKFAST FOLD-OVER

A twist on a Spanish omelette, this is one heavily fortified, high-protein breakfast that's so simple to make and tastes amazing. Also, it's really versatile, so if you want to reduce the fat/calorie content, simply swap out certain ingredients like the feta cheese and mature Cheddar.

1. Spread the green pesto onto one side of the tortilla wrap.

2. Place a frying pan over a medium heat and lightly coat the base with spray light oil. Quickly fry off the onions and baby tomatoes until softened a little then add the egg whites and cook until scrambled, this should only take a few moments.

3. Place the scrambled egg mix onto one half of the pesto-covered wrap then top with the spinach and cheeses. Season with a little salt and pepper then fold the wrap in half to cover the scrambled egg mix.

4. Place the light spread in a large clean frying pan and fry the folded wrap for 2–3 minutes on each side, until golden and crispy.

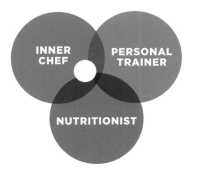

INNER CHEF

PERSONAL TRAINER

NUTRITIONIST

CALORIES 231
PROTEIN 15g
FAT 6g
CARBS 27g
SUGARS 14g

BIRCHER PROTEIN MUESLI POT

SERVES 2

Preparation time: 10 minutes

80g plant-based plain yogurt
50g green apple, grated
½ tsp ground cinnamon
1 scoop (25g) plant-based
   vanilla protein powder
100ml soya milk
1 tbsp maple syrup
30g Ready Brek (or other
   instant oats)
1 tsp golden linseeds
1 tbsp pumpkin seeds
1 tsp raisins
1 tbsp dried cranberries

No need for overnight prepping for this one. Our high-protein Bircher muesli pot is ready in minutes! Made with a creamy, vanilla, yogurt-oat base, mixed with freshly grated apples and sprinkled, seasoned and served with a variety of dried fruit and seeds that give the perfect crunch. Our fridge (or my stomach) is rarely without a pot of this.

1. In a small mixing bowl, whisk together the yogurt, apple, cinnamon, protein powder, soya milk, maple syrup and oats and spoon into two serving bowls.

2. Sprinkle the linseeds, pumpkin seeds, raisins and cranberries on top and enjoy straight away, there's no need to wait!

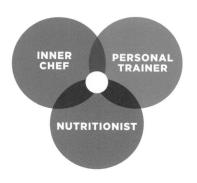

INNER CHEF

PERSONAL TRAINER

NUTRITIONIST

CALORIES 339
PROTEIN 17g
FAT 6g
CARBS 53g
SUGARS 23g

SERVES 5

Preparation time: 10 minutes
Cooking time: 15 minutes

100g (about 3) egg whites
350ml almond milk
2 tsp baking powder
2 scoops (50g) vanilla protein powder
2 tsp vanilla extract
175g plain wholemeal flour
butter-flavour spray oil for cooking

TO SERVE
10 rashers (2 rashers each serving) of streaky bacon
150g (2 tbsp each serving) maple syrup

BACON & MAPLE PROTEIN WAFFLES

Introducing our crispy-on-the-outside and fluffy-and-sweet-on-the-inside smoky bacon and maple protein waffles. It's hard to know just how many of these we've made (and eaten) over the years, but if I had to guess I would say it's in the thousands. It's best to use all the batter while it's fresh, but don't worry if you don't eat all the waffles in one go – you can freeze or refrigerate them. Simply toast them lightly, to crisp and warm them back up when you're ready for round two!

1. Follow the manufacturer's instructions and heat the waffle maker. Preheat the oven to 120°C/100°C fan/gas ½.

2. Using a hand-held electric beater, whisk the egg whites in a clean mixing bowl until they become glossy and stiff peaks form, then set aside.

3. In a separate bowl, whisk all the remaining waffle batter ingredients together until smooth and fully combined.

4. Use a silicone spatula to gently fold the whipped egg whites into the batter mix, taking care not to knock the air bubbles out of the mixture.

5. Coat the waffle maker with a few squirts of the butter-flavoured spray oil then use a large serving spoon or small ladle to pour a portion of batter into the middle of the waffle griddle. Be careful not to go too close to the edges.

6. Cook the waffles for 4–5 minutes or until golden brown. (Follow your waffle-maker instructions as temperatures and timings can vary.) Repeat until all the batter is used, keeping the cooked waffles warm in the low oven.

7. Meanwhile, fry the streaky bacon on medium heat until crisp and place on top of your golden waffles, then drizzle maple syrup over to finish. Enjoy warm.

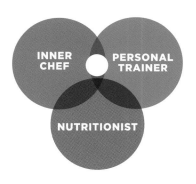

INNER CHEF
PERSONAL TRAINER
NUTRITIONIST

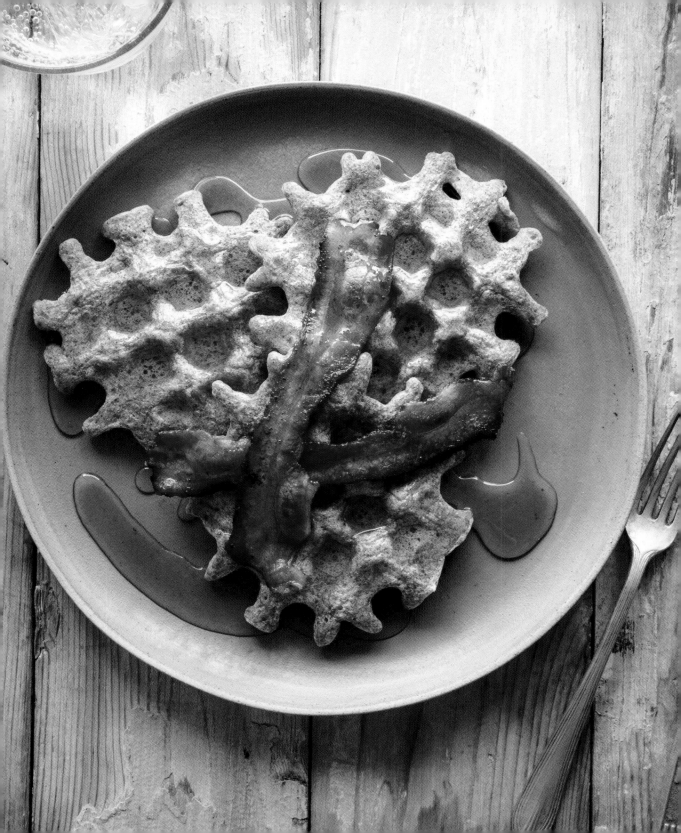

CALORIES 187
PROTEIN 5g
FAT 4g
CARBS 39g
SUGARS 7g

MAKES
16

APPLE CINNAMON STRUDEL ROLLS

Preparation time: 45 minutes +
  proving time
Cooking time: 25 minutes

FOR THE DOUGH
2½ tsp active dry yeast
40g Flora Light spread
  (or other light spread)
50g zero-calorie granulated
  white sugar replacer
600g strong white
  bread flour
½ tsp salt
spray light oil for greasing

FOR THE FILLING
900g Bramley, Granny Smith,
  Pink Lady, Jazz, Braeburn
  or other firm apples
1 tbsp ground cinnamon
30g Flora Light spread
  (or other light spread)
100g zero-calorie granulated
  white sugar replacer

FOR THE GLAZE
30g Flora Light spread
  (or other light spread)
115g Philadelphia Lightest
  cream cheese (or other
  low-fat cream cheese)
125g zero-calorie powdered
  icing sugar replacer
1 tsp vanilla bean paste

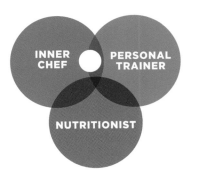

A healthy alternative that's been designed to combat cravings, these can be eaten any time of the day, but a freshly baked tray never lasts long in our house. Crispy on the outside, but soft, light and fluffy on the inside. The vanilla glaze, made with a low-fat cream cheese, is brilliantly complimented by the fruity apple and cinnamon filling. See the photo on the next page.

1. Start making the dough by mixing the yeast with 100ml of warm water in a small bowl and leave for 10 minutes until it is frothy and bubbly.

2. Using a stand mixer with a whisk attachment, mix together 180ml of hot water, the light spread and the sweetener until the spread has melted into the water. Leave to cool slightly before adding 400g of the bread flour and the salt and mix to bind the ingredients. (If you don't have a stand mixer use a large bowl and a wooden spoon instead.)

3. Pour the yeast into the mixture along with the remaining bread flour and mix until fully combined.

4. Use a dough hook to knead the dough until it is smooth in texture then take the dough out of the bowl and knead a few times by hand to create a nice smooth ball. (If you don't have a stand mixer knead by hand for 5–10 minutes instead, until the dough is smooth.)

5. Place the kneaded dough back into the mixing bowl, cover with a clean tea towel and leave in a warm place for 1 hour to prove, until doubled in size.

6. While the dough is proving, prepare the filling. Peel, core and roughly chop the apples into 1-cm chunks and place into a medium saucepan with the cinnamon. Place the saucepan over a medium heat and cook the apples, stirring often, until they have softened a little but still retain their shape. This should take around 10 minutes. Turn off the heat and set aside to cool.

7. After the dough has completed its first rise, cut it in half and roll into a rectangular shape measuring 50 x 30cm, making sure the surface is well floured as you do not want it to stick at all.

8. Melt 30g of the spread and lightly brush the surface of the rolled-out dough with half of the melted spread. Sprinkle half of the granulated sweetener on the surface of the dough then spoon half the apple cinnamon mixture on top.

9. Roll the dough up from the shorter side, trying to keep the roll tight without stretching it. Cut a little bit off both ends to even the roll up then cut into 8 rolls and place into a lightly greased 20-cm round cake tin. Leave in a warm place to prove for another half an hour.

10. Repeat this process with the remaining half of the dough.

11. Preheat the oven to 170°C/150°C fan/gas 3.

12. When both tins of rolls have had their second prove, bake them in the preheated oven for 20–25 minutes until the surface of the cinnamon rolls are golden brown. Leave to cool a little while you prepare the glaze.

13. To make the glaze, melt the spread and place into a mixing bowl with the remainder of the glaze ingredients and beat together until smooth.

14. Once both trays of cinnamon buns have cooled a little, spread the glaze over both trays of rolls and either leave to cool completely or dig in while they are still warm.

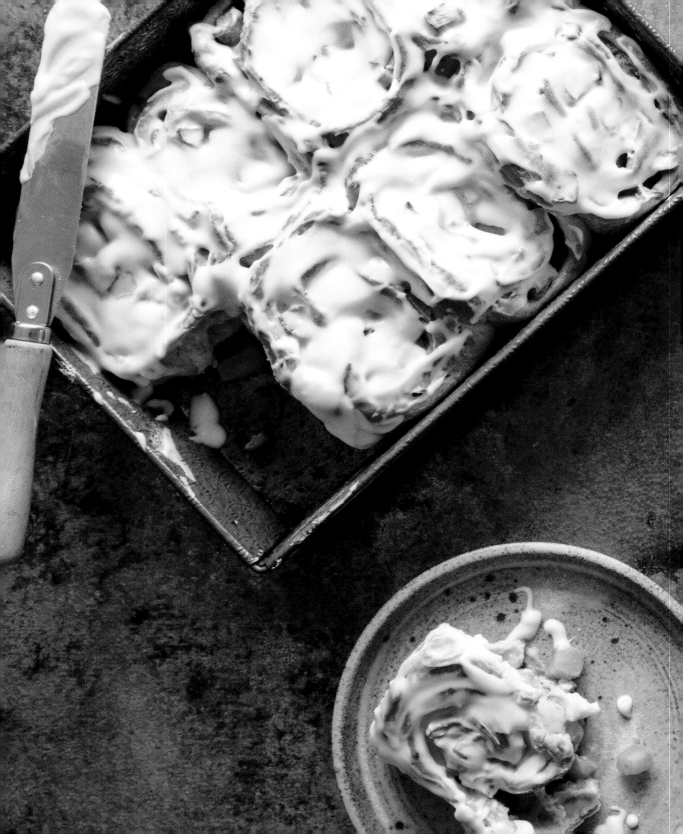

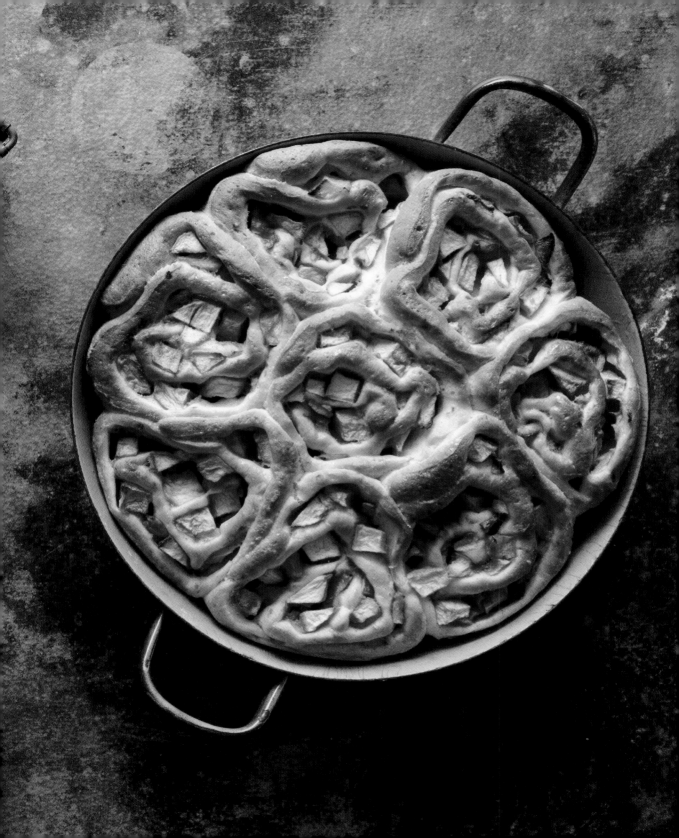

Lunch

The lunch menu in this book is legendary. It contains some of the strongest sandwiches, salads and stir-fry recipes your kitchen cupboards have ever seen and a secret homemade burger sauce that can be used on anything and everything. Seasoned to perfection and packed with protein, basically, you won't just like lunchtime … you will love it!

SAFFRON & LEMON CHICKEN JOOJEH KEBABS

SERVES 2

Preparation time: 15 minutes +
    24 hours marinating
Cooking time: 15 minutes

¼ tsp saffron threads
200g 0%-fat Greek yogurt
juice of 1 lemon
½ white onion, thinly sliced
2 chicken breasts, chopped into
    4-cm pieces
sea salt and freshly ground
    black pepper
2 flatbreads (optional)

FOR THE SALAD
100g baby leaf salad
100g cucumber, diced
100g baby plum tomatoes,
    halved
1 yellow pepper, sliced
½ white onion, thinly sliced
1 tbsp lemon juice

A Persian joojeh kebab! If you're looking for a less-carby meal choice, this is such a go-to. Fresh and creamy with a delicate saffron and lemon flavour, combined with a zingy salad and an optional fluffy flatbread.

1. First, bloom the saffron. Grind the threads with the back of a spoon and place in a cup with 2 tablespoons of boiling water. Leave to steep for 10 minutes, until the flavour and colour of the saffron have infused into the water.

2. In a large mixing bowl, mix the yogurt, bloomed saffron, lemon juice and onion along with a good pinch of salt. Mix in the chicken and stir everything together. Cover the bowl and place in the fridge for 24 hours. The longer you leave the mixture to marinate the more the flavours will develop. (If you're short on time a few hours will be okay.)

3. Take the marinated chicken out of the fridge and leave to come to room temperature for 30 minutes before you are ready to cook.

4. Thread the marinated chicken onto skewers and place on a hot griddle pan. Cook the skewers for 2–3 minutes on each side until they are cooked through and have some delicious char marks.

5. Prepare the salad by mixing all the ingredients in a bowl, ensuring the lemon juice has coated everything. Season to taste with salt and pepper. Serve alongside your kebabs with a flatbread, if you like.

Tip: If you are using bamboo skewers make sure you soak them in water for at least half an hour before you thread the chicken onto them. This helps make sure they don't burn during cooking. This recipe would also work really well on a barbecue.

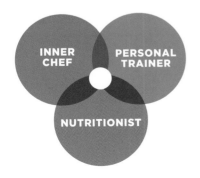

INNER CHEF

PERSONAL TRAINER

NUTRITIONIST

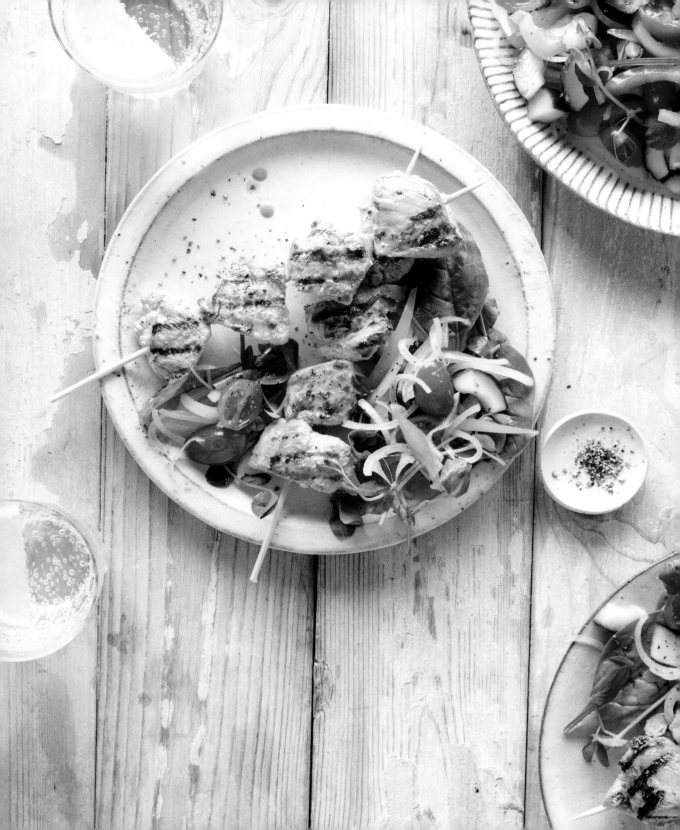

CALORIES 439
PROTEIN 44g
FAT 8g
CARBS 41g
SUGARS 16g

Preparation time: 10 minutes
Cooking time: 10 minutes

150g wholewheat couscous
1 red onion, thinly sliced
1 tbsp zero-calorie granulated
   white sugar replacer
1 tbsp balsamic vinegar
30g/1 bunch fresh coriander
   leaves, roughly chopped
50g spinach leaves
2 skinless chicken breasts
40g pomegranate seeds
20g flaked almonds
spray light oil for cooking

FOR THE POMEGRANATE DRESSING
1 tbsp clear honey
2 tbsp pomegranate molasses
2 tbsp cold water

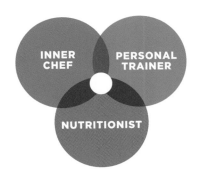

GRILLED CHICKEN, POMEGRANATE & ALMOND SALAD

SERVES 2

A sweet couscous salad, tossed with caramelised onions and drenched in pomegranate dressing with grilled chicken pieces on top. This one would be perfect to prepare in advance for an easy, relaxed lunch with friends, and the chicken can be cooked on a barbecue if you want to dine al fresco!

1. Place the couscous in a large salad bowl and pour over 350ml of boiling water. Stir and set aside to absorb the water, then allow it to cool completely.

2. Coat the base of a small frying pan with spray light oil and fry the onions over a medium heat until soft. Add the sweetener and balsamic vinegar, and simmer for a further 3 minutes, stirring well to ensure the onions are well coated. Add the cooked onions to the couscous along with the coriander and spinach leaves.

3. To make the dressing, mix together the honey, pomegranate molasses and water in a small bowl. Pour over the couscous salad and mix everything together. If you are preparing in advance, place the salad in the fridge, then remove the salad and the raw chicken from the fridge 30 minutes before cooking the chicken and serving to bring them up to room temperature.

4. Heat a griddle pan over a medium-high heat, spray the chicken breasts with a little spray light oil and cook for 4–5 minutes on each side until the outside has some char marks and the inside is thoroughly cooked (the meat should have no hint of pinkness and the juices should run clear when gently pressed). If you prefer, you can cook the chicken breasts on a preheated barbecue, using a meat thermometer to check they are cooked through (insert the probe into the middle of the thickest part of the breast, it should read at least 70°C).

5. Slice the chicken breasts into thin strips and place on top of the salad before finally sprinkling over the pomegranate seeds and almonds for extra crunch.

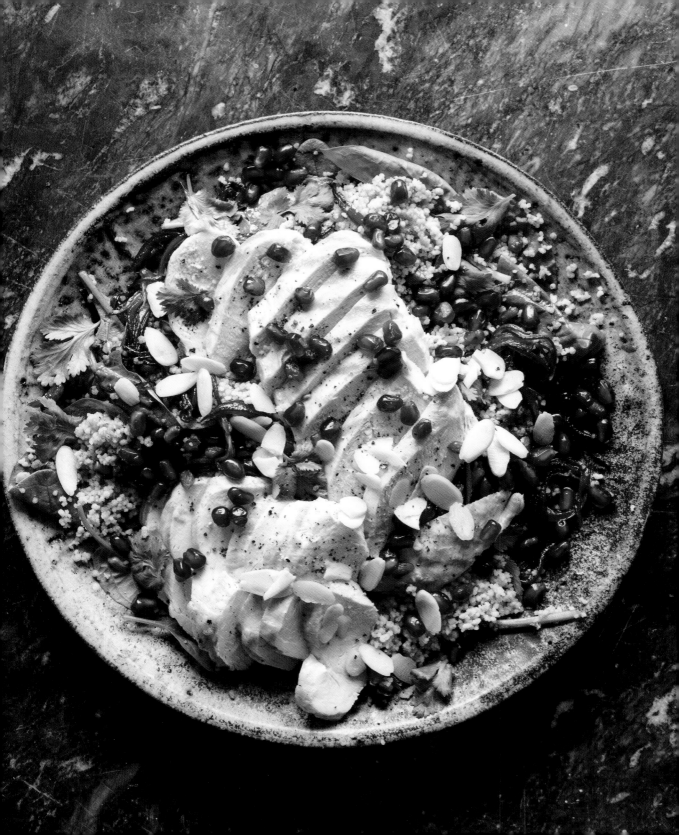

CALORIES 428
PROTEIN 42g
FAT 7g
CARBS 50g
SUGARS 19g

SERVES
5

TURKEY BURGERS WITH SPECIAL BURGER SAUCE

Preparation time: 15 minutes
Cooking time: 15 minutes

FOR THE BURGER PATTIES
500g turkey mince
1 red onion, finely diced
3 spring onions, finely chopped
½ tsp garlic powder
1 tsp onion powder
15g/½ bunch fresh parsley,
    finely chopped
1 egg
30g panko breadcrumbs
sea salt and freshly ground
    black pepper
spray light oil for cooking

FOR THE BURGER SAUCE
1 shallot, finely chopped
200g pickled gherkins
¼ tsp mustard powder
½ tsp ground paprika
½ tsp tomato purée
½ tsp onion powder
¼ tsp garlic powder
1 tbsp wholegrain mustard
1 tsp turmeric
2 tbsp mirin
2 tbsp gherkin water
1 tbsp zero-calorie granulated
    white sugar replacer
3 tbsp Lighter than Light
    mayonnaise

Burger sauce is always used in this house, and if Hester doesn't hide the bottle half of it will be gone in one sitting! So it was only fitting to make a cleaner version for our turkey burgers. This is a low-fat alternative burger, swapping red meat for leaner white meat and an oily sauce for a thicker, chutney-style burger sauce with the signature gherkin punch! This recipe makes more burger sauce than you will need, but any leftovers can be kept in an airtight container in the fridge for several days.

TO SERVE
5 brioche buns
80g gem lettuce, sliced
50g sliced gherkins
3 salad tomatoes, sliced

1. In a mixing bowl, knead together the burger patty ingredients along with a good pinch of salt and pepper, and shape the mixture into five patties, each about the size of your palm.

2. Heat a large frying pan over a medium heat and cover the base with spray light oil. Fry the burger patties for 4–5 minutes on each side until golden brown and cooked through.

3. To make the burger sauce, lightly fry the shallot then place in a blender with the remainder of the burger sauce ingredients and blitz until smooth and runny.

4. Build your burger by placing the lettuce on the base of the brioche bun, followed by the cooked patty, then layers of gherkin and tomato. Drizzle with the burger sauce and finally close the burger with the brioche top.

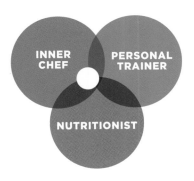

INNER CHEF
PERSONAL TRAINER
NUTRITIONIST

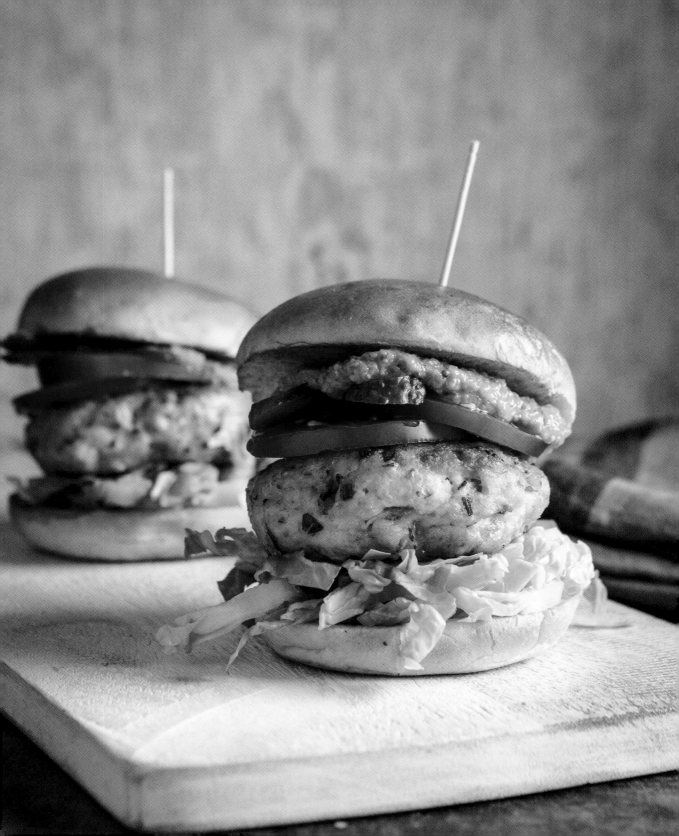

SERVES 2

POMEGRANATE PORK WITH BEETROOT, FETA & CUCUMBER SALAD

Preparation time: 10 minutes
Cooking time: 20–25 minutes

4 pork chops
spray light oil for cooking

FOR THE POMEGRANATE
   DRESSING
1½ tbsp pomegranate molasses
2 tbsp pomegranate juice
1 tbsp balsamic vinegar
½ tbsp clear honey

FOR THE BEETROOT SALAD
50g spinach leaves
30g rocket leaves
250g cucumber, diced
50g feta cheese, chopped into
   1-cm chunks
100g cooked beetroot (not
   pickled), chopped into
   1-cm chunks
sea salt and freshly ground
   black pepper

I think we can agree that this is the simplest, most heart-warming salad to make. With every mouthful of tender pork comes a rich, deep, pomegranate and balsamic flavour with a hit of saltiness coming through from the feta cheese.

1. Preheat the oven to 200°C/180°C fan/gas 6.

2. Place the pork chops on a lightly oiled baking tray and cook in the preheated oven for 20 minutes, turning them halfway through the cooking time. (Keep an eye on your pork chops as the cooking time will depend a little on how thick the chops are. They are done when their juices run clear.)

3. In a small bowl mix together all the dressing ingredients and set aside.

4. Place the spinach, rocket and cucumber in a large salad bowl, season with salt and pepper and pour over most of the pomegranate dressing. Mix well.

5. To serve, top the salad with the feta cheese and beetroot chunks, place the pork chops on top, and finish with a drizzle of the remaining pomegranate dressing.

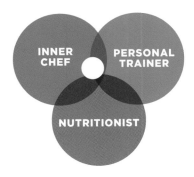

INNER CHEF · PERSONAL TRAINER · NUTRITIONIST

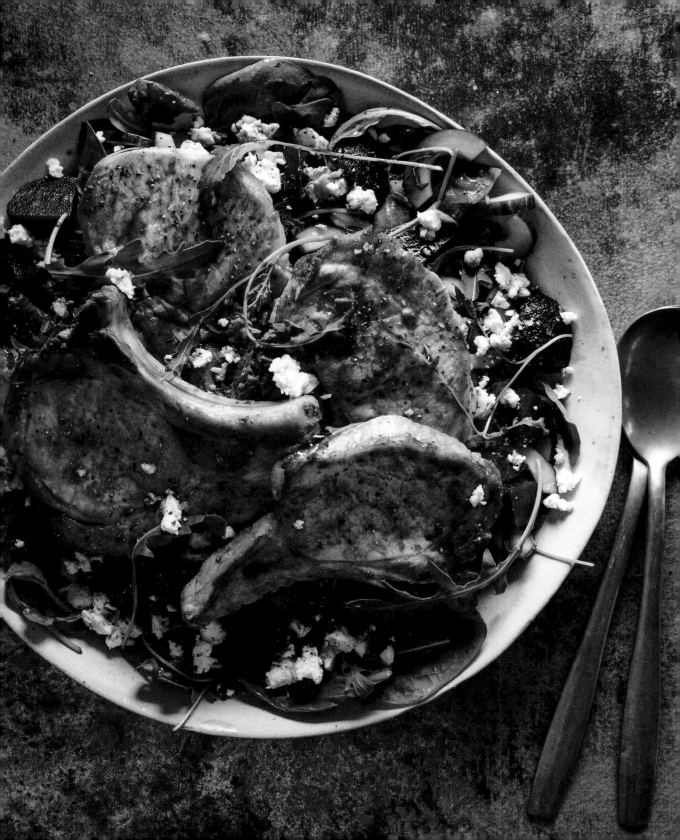

CALORIES 522
PROTEIN 53g
FAT 12g
CARBS 49g
SUGARS 3g

CRISPY CHICKEN STRIPS & KFC-STYLE GRAVY

SERVES 2

Preparation time: 20 minutes
Cooking time: 20 minutes

1 tsp dried basil
1 tsp dried thyme
1 tbsp smoked paprika
2 tsp ground white pepper
1 tsp garlic powder
1 tsp onion powder
¼ tsp mustard powder
½ tsp ground ginger
50g plain white flour
2 eggs, beaten
60g panko breadcrumbs
2 chicken breasts, cut into
    1.5-cm strips
sea salt and freshly ground
    black pepper
spray light oil for cooking

FOR THE GRAVY DIPPING SAUCE
½ chicken stock cube
½ beef stock cube
1 tbsp plain flour
½ tsp onion powder
½ tsp garlic powder
¼ tsp ground white pepper

This is such a simple but tasty lunch. There's no need to spend the calories on a takeaway when you can fakeaway at home. We normally pair this with the Shirazi Salad (see page 130) to add a bit of greenery. I always ask for more of these, I don't think anyone could ever get enough!

1. Preheat the oven to 200°C/180°C fan/gas 6 and line a baking tray with parchment paper.

2. In a large bowl, mix together the herbs, spices, flour and a good pinch each of salt and pepper. Prepare two more bowls, one with the beaten eggs and one with the panko breadcrumbs.

3. Take each strip of chicken and dip it first into the flour and herb mix, then into the egg (being careful to gently shake off any excess egg), then finally coat the seasoned chicken strips in the panko breadcrumbs.

4. Place the chicken pieces on the baking tray and spray with oil.

5. Bake the chicken strips in the oven for 20 minutes, turning them halfway through the cooking time and spraying again with oil.

6. While the chicken is cooking, make the gravy. In a jug, mix together 500ml of boiling water and the stock cubes followed by the rest of the gravy ingredients. Use a small whisk or stick blender to make sure there are no lumps of flour. Place in a small saucepan and bring to the boil while stirring all the while. The flour should thicken the gravy slightly and give it the perfect consistency for dipping.

7. Pour the gravy into two small bowls or ramekins and serve alongside the chicken strips, with a green salad.

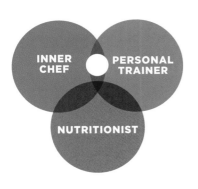

INNER CHEF

PERSONAL TRAINER

NUTRITIONIST

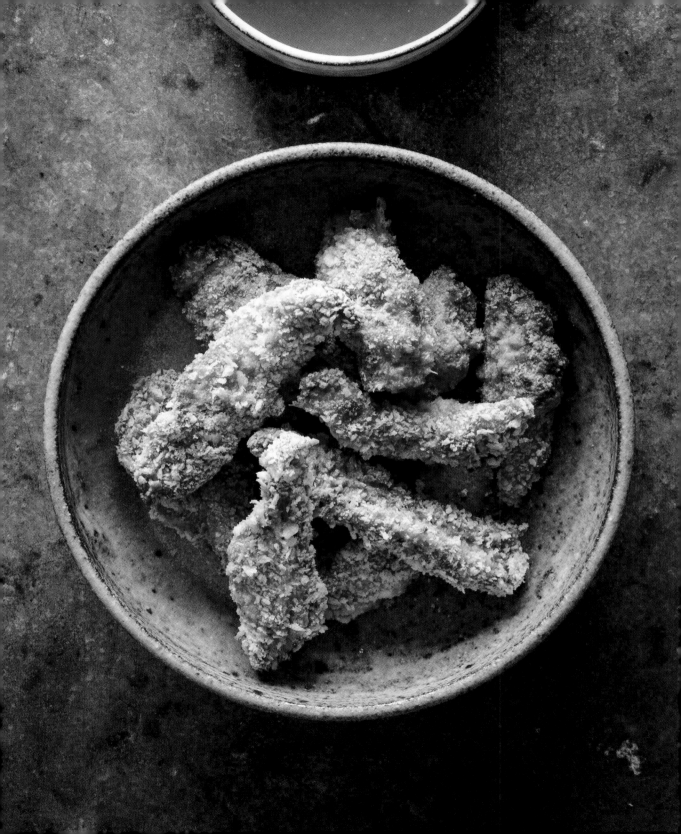

CALORIES 381
PROTEIN 29g
FAT 21g
CARBS 19g
SUGARS 12g

SERVES 2

OVEN-BAKED SWEET CHILLI SALMON & SESAME SALAD BOWL

Preparation time: 15 minutes
Cooking time: 20 minutes

2 salmon fillets
sea salt and freshly ground
   black pepper

FOR THE SALAD
80g carrot, coarsely grated
100g white cabbage, finely
   grated
3 spring onions, chopped
1 yellow pepper, thinly sliced
½ cucumber, julienned
20g cashew nuts
10g/⅓ bunch fresh coriander,
   roughly chopped
1 tbsp sesame oil

FOR THE DRESSING
1 tsp garlic purée
140g zero-calorie granulated
   white sugar replacer
1 tsp ginger purée
2 tsp chilli purée
4 tbsp light soy sauce
100ml boiling water
2 tbsp apple cider vinegar
2 tsp arrowroot

A meaty, perfectly oven-baked salmon fillet, lying on a bed of sweetly grated sesame salad, with lashings of sweet chilli dressing.

1. Preheat the oven to 180°C/160°C fan/gas 4.

2. Place the salmon fillets in an aluminium foil parcel, with a pinch each of salt and pepper, and bake in the oven for 20 minutes.

3. Meanwhile, prepare the salad by mixing all the ingredients together in a large mixing bowl.

4. Next make the sweet chilli dressing by mixing all the ingredients, apart from the arrowroot, together in a small saucepan. Place the arrowroot in a separate small bowl with 4 tablespoons of cold water and mix together until there are no lumps.

5. Five minutes before the end of the salmon cooking time, place the sweet chilli dressing ingredients, including the arrowroot solution, over a medium heat and pour in 100ml of boiling water. Stir continuously until the sauce is simmering and has thickened slightly, then immediately take off the heat.

6. Serve the crunchy root salad in a pasta bowl, ensuring the sesame oil coats everything. Place the baked salmon on top and pour over the sweet chilli dressing. Finish by garnishing with a sprinkle of sesame seeds, if you like.

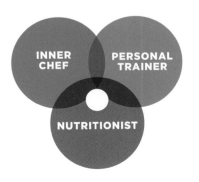

INNER CHEF
PERSONAL TRAINER
NUTRITIONIST

CALORIES 417
PROTEIN 9g
FAT 18g
CARBS 52g
SUGARS 38g

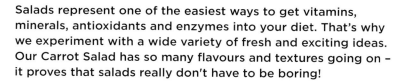

CARROT SALAD

SERVES 2

Preparation time: 20 minutes
Cooking time: 10 minutes

100g bulgur wheat
250g carrots, grated
100g edamame beans
30g/1 bunch fresh coriander
  leaves, roughly chopped
15g/½ bunch fresh mint, roughly
  chopped
50g dried cranberries

FOR THE DRESSING
1 tsp apple cider vinegar
2 tbsp rice vinegar
2 tbsp clear honey
2 tbsp sesame seed oil

Salads represent one of the easiest ways to get vitamins, minerals, antioxidants and enzymes into your diet. That's why we experiment with a wide variety of fresh and exciting ideas. Our Carrot Salad has so many flavours and textures going on – it proves that salads really don't have to be boring!

1. Place the bulgur wheat in a sieve and rinse with cold water until the water runs clear. Place in a saucepan with 300ml of just-boiled water, bring back to the boil then turn down the heat to simmer and cook for 10 minutes, until the bulgur wheat is just tender. (Add a little more water if the bottom of the pan starts to catch.) Once cooked, drain any remaining water from the pan and set aside to cool completely.

2. In a large salad bowl add the grated carrots, edamame beans, coriander, mint and cranberries along with the cooled bulgur wheat and stir everything together.

3. To make the dressing, mix all the ingredients together in small bowl and pour over the carrot salad. Mix together thoroughly to coat the salad with the dressing.

4. You can enjoy this salad straight away, but if you leave it to sit for an hour or two, the coriander and mint infuse into the bulgur wheat a little more, adding even more depth of flavour.

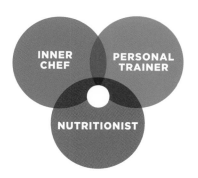

INNER CHEF
PERSONAL TRAINER
NUTRITIONIST

CALORIES 408
PROTEIN 48g
FAT 12g
CARBS 23g
SUGARS 18g

FIRECRACKER CHICKEN STIR-FRY

Preparation time: 10 minutes
Cooking time: 20 minutes

2 skinless chicken breasts, chopped into 3-cm chunks
160g kimchi (Korean pickled cabbage)
50g edamame beans, fresh or frozen
50g carrot, finely grated
150g beansprouts
160g sugar snaps
3 spring onions, finely sliced
80g romaine lettuce leaves, thinly shredded
10g/⅓ bunch fresh coriander leaves, roughly chopped
spray light oil for cooking

FOR THE MISO SESAME DRESSING
1 tsp white miso paste
1 tbsp light soy sauce
1 tsp rice vinegar
2 tbsp lime juice
1 tbsp clear honey
1 tsp ginger purée
1 tsp sesame seed oil

I love Firecracker Chicken, but have to confess my taste buds can't handle the spice and heat that comes from the dish when it's in its original, traditional form. Which is exactly why we perfected a healthy, homemade version so we could tweak, tailor and tame the chilli content whilst keeping the same taste, texture and flavour. The result is a nutrient-dense, protein-packed recipe that you can eat over and over again.

1. Place the chicken in a medium bowl and mix in the kimchi. Cover the bowl and place in the fridge to marinate for at least 4 hours but preferably overnight.

2. To make the miso sesame dressing, whisk together all the dressing ingredients in a small bowl and set aside.

3. Coat the base of a large frying pan with spray light oil and fry the chicken and kimchi over a medium heat for 10–15 minutes, until the chicken is cooked through. If your edamame beans are frozen, cook them in the pan at the same time.

4. When the chicken is cooked, add the edamame beans, if you have not done so already, the carrot, beansprouts, sugar snaps and spring onions to the pan and stir-fry with the chicken for a few minutes to heat through the vegetables.

5. Finally, stir in the shredded lettuce and remove from the heat. Divide into two bowls, pour over the dressing and scatter over the coriander.

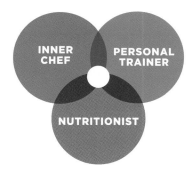

INNER CHEF
PERSONAL TRAINER
NUTRITIONIST

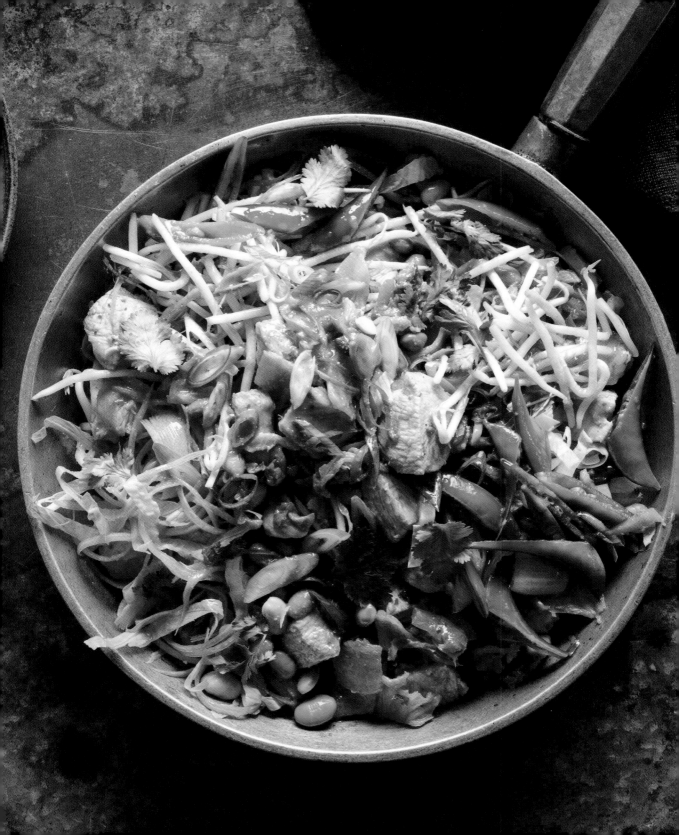

CALORIES 464
PROTEIN 29g
FAT 7g
CARBS 65g
SUGARS 8g

Preparation time: 15 minutes
Cooking time: 15 minutes

15g white flour
15g panko breadcrumbs
1 egg, beaten
1 white cod loin fillet
1 panini roll
handful of rocket
sea salt and freshly ground
    black pepper
spray light oil for cooking

FOR THE CELERIAC &
    CAPER REMOULADE
80g celeriac, coarsely grated
15g capers
40g Lighter than Light
    mayonnaise
½ tbsp lemon juice
1 tsp wholegrain mustard

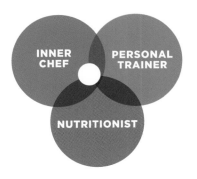

FISH FINGER SANDWICH WITH CELERIAC & CAPER REMOULADE

SERVES 1

This is what you call a clean sandwich. It naturally contains 29g of protein. A white, meaty fish fillet in golden-brown crispy breadcrumbs, placed on a fresh leaf salad and topped with a light and zingy celeriac and caper remoulade. Yes, this is quite a carb-heavy meal. However, depending on your goals and when you eat a meal like this, it could be perfect for you. To make it less carb-heavy, substitute the panini for extra green salad.

1. Preheat the oven to 200°C/180°C fan/gas 6 and line a baking tray with parchment paper.

2. Start by breading the cod fillet. Prepare one bowl with the flour and season with salt and pepper. Prepare another bowl with the panko breadcrumbs and a third bowl with the beaten egg. Pat the fish dry with a piece of kitchen towel then dip the cod loin into the seasoned flour, then the egg (being careful to gently shake off any excess egg), then in the breadcrumbs. Gently press the fish into the crumbs to make sure the fillet is well coated.

3. Place the cod fillet on the lined baking tray, spray with oil then bake for 12–15 minutes until the cod is just cooked and golden brown.

4. Meanwhile, make the remoulade by mixing the celeriac, capers, mayonnaise, lemon juice, mustard and a good pinch of pepper together in a mixing bowl. Set aside until the fish has cooked.

5. Warm the panini by slicing it in half and placing it in the oven for a few minutes towards the end of the fish cooking time.

6. Assemble the sandwich by spooning the remoulade on the bottom half of the panini, followed by the rocket. Place the crispy fish fillet on top and pop on the panini top.

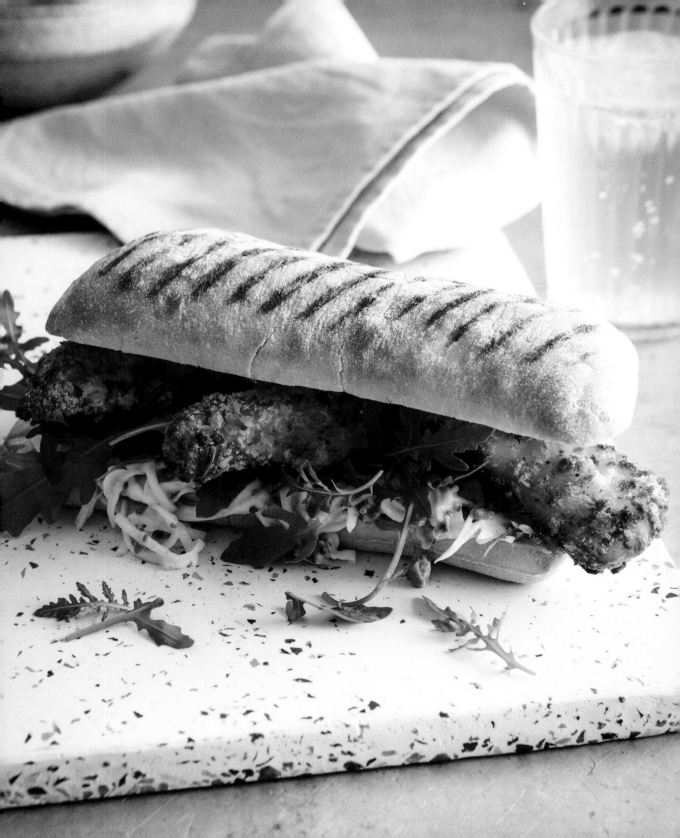

CALORIES 500
PROTEIN 52g
FAT 17g
CARBS 32g
SUGARS 13g

SERVES 4

Preparation time: 20 minutes
Cooking time: 20 minutes

4 chicken breasts
3 tbsp plain flour
2 eggs, beaten
60g panko breadcrumbs

FOR THE KATSU SAUCE
1 onion, finely chopped
170g carrots, grated
½ tsp ginger purée
½ tsp garlic purée
2 tsp light soya sauce
250ml chicken stock
1½ tsp ground cumin
2 tbsp curry powder
1 tsp turmeric
1 tbsp agave syrup
150ml light coconut milk

FOR THE SALAD
20g/⅔ bunch fresh coriander,
   chopped
200g edamame beans
200g carrots, grated
200g cucumber, sliced
200g gem lettuce, sliced
sesame seeds, for sprinkling

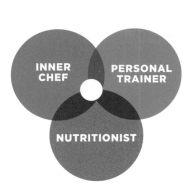

INNER CHEF   PERSONAL TRAINER   NUTRITIONIST

CHICKEN KATSU CURRY

A silky Katsu curry sauce ... not too hot and not too sweet, poured on top of a crispy, golden-brown, tender chicken breast on a bed of freshly prepared salad. Definitely a lunchtime treat to look forward to.

1. Preheat the oven to 200°C/180°C fan/gas 6 and line a baking tray with parchment paper.

2. Cover the chicken breasts with a large piece of cling film and use a rolling pin to tap them until they are slightly flattened.

3. Place the flour in one bowl, the beaten eggs in another and the panko breadcrumbs in a third. Piece by piece, place the chicken in the flour, then the egg, then the panko, making sure to coat the chicken thoroughly with each ingredient and really pressing the breadcrumbs on.

4. Place the chicken on the lined baking tray and cook in the oven for 20 minutes until golden brown and cooked through.

5. Meanwhile, lightly fry the onion and grated carrots in some spray light oil over a medium heat until the onions are translucent. Place in a blender along with the remainder of the katsu sauce ingredients and blend until smooth. Pour the katsu sauce back into the frying pan and bring to a simmer for 5 minutes until heated through and slightly thickened.

6. Make the salad by tossing all the salad ingredients together.

7. Place the crispy chicken on one side of a bowl and pour over the katsu curry sauce. Place the salad on the other side of the bowl and finish with a sprinkle of sesame seeds.

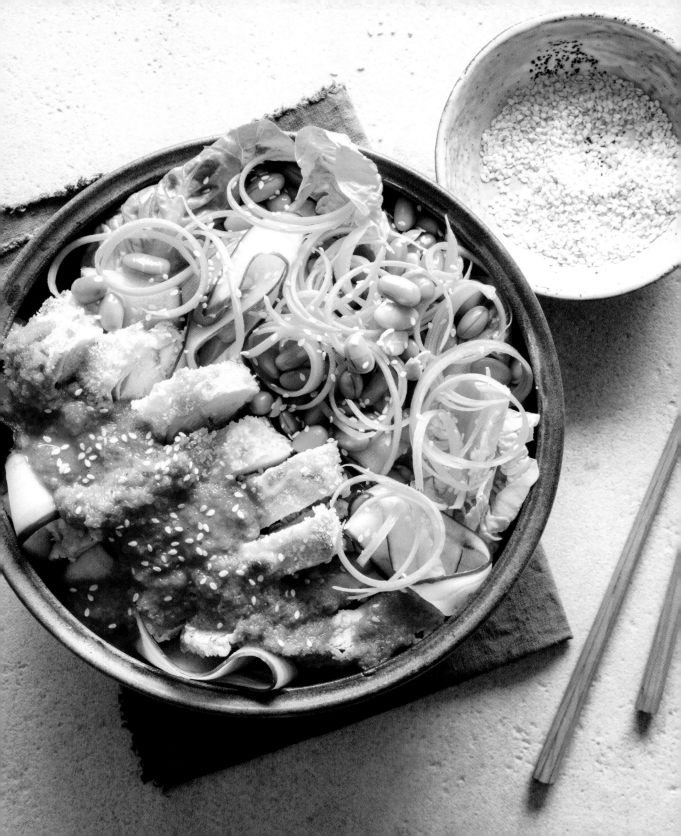

CALORIES 456
PROTEIN 43g
FAT 20g
CARBS 26g
SUGARS 21g

Preparation time: 5 minutes
Cooking time: 50 minutes

6 large chicken wings
125g fresh mango, peeled
   and chopped
3 tbsp maple syrup
juice of 1 lime

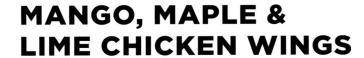

MANGO, MAPLE & LIME CHICKEN WINGS

SERVES 2

A fruity lunch option that you can pair with almost anything, whether a fresh salad, homemade slaw or some stir-fried vegetables.

1. Preheat the oven to 200°C/180°C fan/gas 6 and line a baking tray with parchment paper.

2. Place the chicken wings on the lined baking tray and cook in the oven for 30 minutes.

3. Meanwhile, blitz the mango, maple syrup and lime juice together in a blender.

4. After 30 minutes of cooking time, pour the glaze over the chicken wings and bake for a further 20 minutes, turning the chicken halfway through the final cooking time so each side has a chance to get crispy.

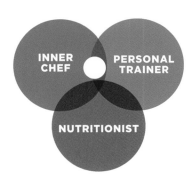

INNER CHEF

PERSONAL TRAINER

NUTRITIONIST

CALORIES 259
PROTEIN 36g
FAT 9g
CARBS 8g
SUGARS 5g

SERVES 2

LEMONY GARLIC-BAKED WHITE FISH

Preparation time: 10 minutes
Cooking time: 15 minutes

250g/2 cod fillets
125g asparagus
100g fine green beans
100g mangetout

FOR THE LEMON BUTTER SAUCE
50g Flora Light spread (or
    other light spread)
juice of 1 lemon
½ tsp garlic purée
1 tsp dried dill
1 tsp dried thyme
8g/¼ bunch fresh parsley,
    finely chopped

This dish is perfect if you're wanting a low-calorie, high-protein lunch. However, it also pairs really well with a few boiled new potatoes smothered in garlic butter or a creamy mash, if you're feeling the need for a more generous serving of carbs, depending on your goals.

1. Preheat the oven to 200°C/180°C fan/gas 6 and line a baking tray with parchment paper.

2. Place the cod, asparagus, green beans and mangetout on the lined baking tray and set aside.

3. Heat a small saucepan over a medium heat and melt the light spread together with the lemon juice, garlic purée, dill, thyme and parsley. As soon as the spread has melted, stir everything together and pour the sauce over the cod and green vegetables.

4. Place in the oven and bake for 15 minutes until the cod is cooked through and the greens have softened slightly but crisped up a little on the edges.

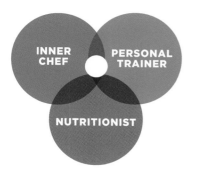

INNER CHEF · PERSONAL TRAINER · NUTRITIONIST

BRESAOLA TOASTY

CALORIES 438
PROTEIN 27g
FAT 18g
CARBS 41g
SUGARS 3g

SERVES
1

Preparation time: 5 minutes
Cooking time: 5 minutes

30g reduced-fat green pesto
2 slices sourdough
35g bresaola (or serrano ham)
15g Parmesan cheese, finely
    grated
a large handful of bistro salad
20g Flora light spread (or other
    light spread)
freshly ground black pepper

Probably the richest-tasting toasty ever, with smoky cured bresaola slices, a strong green pesto kick, a hit of grated Parmesan, and a colourful bistro salad sandwiched between two toasted sourdough slices. We made these in the summer every day and sat in the conservatory munching on our sandwiches in the sun.

1. Spread the pesto over the slices of sourdough.

2. Lay the bresaola on top of the pesto on one of the slices of bread, followed by the Parmesan, a good pinch of black pepper and the bistro salad. Then top with the second piece of sourdough.

3. Butter the top and the underside of the sandwich with the spread and place in a frying pan over a medium heat. Cook for a few minutes on each side until golden brown.

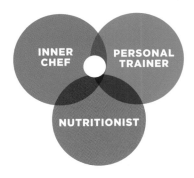

INNER CHEF
PERSONAL TRAINER
NUTRITIONIST

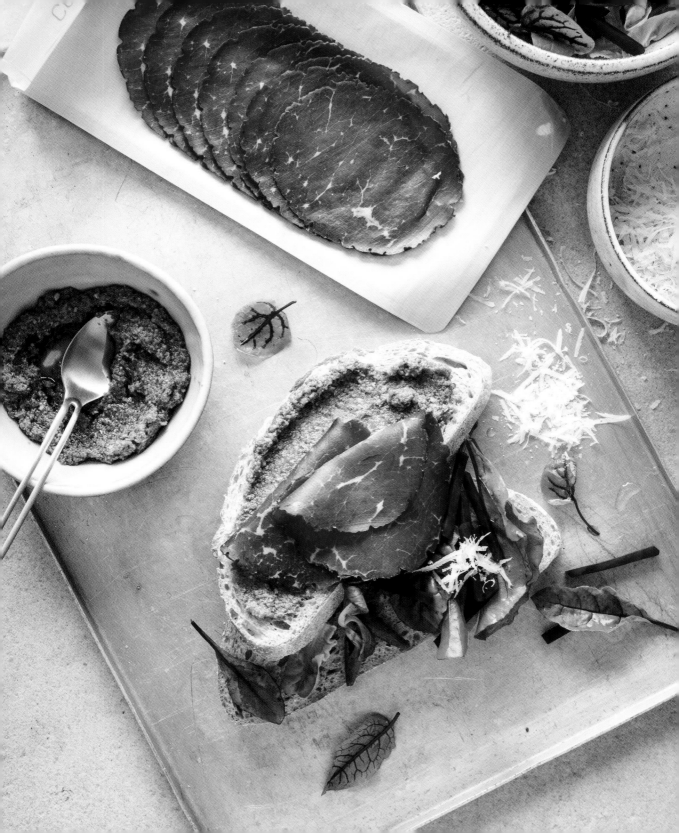

SUPER NUTTY SALAD

SERVES 2

Preparation time: 15 minutes
Cooking time: 15 minutes

100g tricolour quinoa
(a mix of white, red and black
quinoa)
40g broccoli, chopped into tiny
pieces
60g tinned black-eyed peas,
drained and rinsed
10g pistachios
15g almonds
15g peanuts
10g cashew nuts
15g pumpkin seeds
30g edamame beans
30g peas
50g carrot, chopped into
tiny pieces

FOR THE GINGER AND SOY
DRESSING
1 tbsp rice vinegar
3 tbsp pomegranate juice
juice from 1 lime
2 tsp ginger purée
½ tsp garlic purée
15g fresh coriander,
finely chopped
2 tsp light soy sauce

Packed with protein and good fats, we could just keep eating and eating this salad! There are so many textures and flavours. I know there are quite a few ingredients to this recipe but it's quick to put together and if you make a big batch you could have lunch sorted for several days.

1. Bring 300ml of water to the boil in a large saucepan over a high heat and rinse the quinoa thoroughly under running water until the water runs clear.

2. Add the quinoa to the boiling water, stir and cover with a lid. Reduce the heat and simmer for 15 minutes, adding the broccoli and black-eyed peas for the last few minutes of the cooking time. Drain well and leave to cool then fluff up with a fork.

3. Mix the remainder of the salad ingredients into the quinoa, broccoli and black-eyed pea mix, making sure the nuts are spread evenly to get some crunch with every bite.

4. Prepare the dressing by mixing all the ingredients together in a small bowl. Pour the dressing on top of the salad and give everything a good stir to coat. This salad will keep, covered, in the fridge for 2 days.

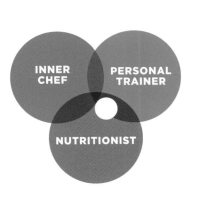

INNER CHEF
PERSONAL TRAINER
NUTRITIONIST

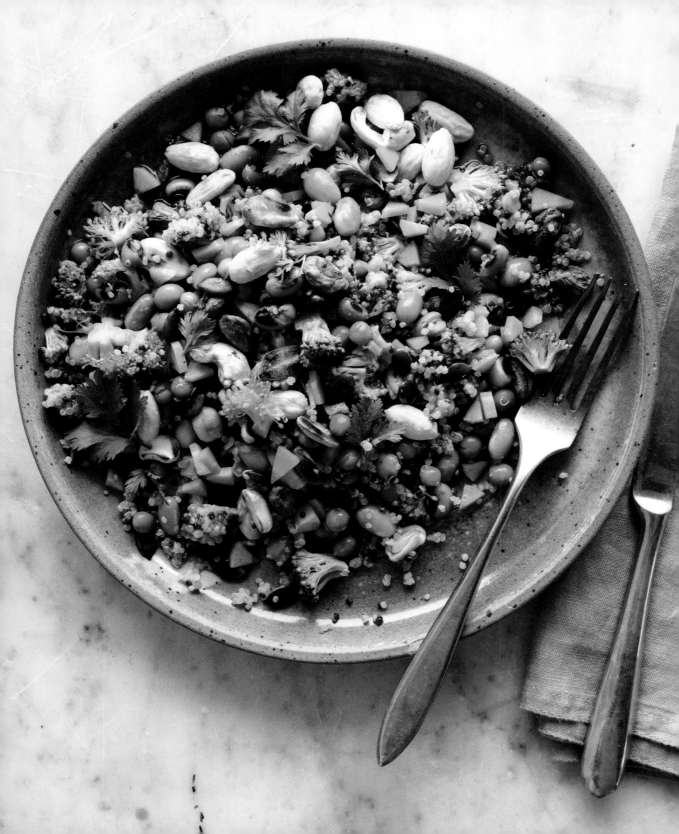

CALORIES 479
PROTEIN 38g
FAT 15g
CARBS 47g
SUGARS 21g

SERVES 2

SHREDDED HOISIN DUCK BURGER

Preparation time: 10 minutes +
    15 minutes resting
Cooking time: 30 minutes

½ tsp Chinese five spice
2 duck breasts
100g carrot, coarsely grated
2 spring onions, sliced
1 red onion, finely chopped
3 tbsp light soy sauce
2 tbsp hoisin sauce
spray light oil for cooking

TO SERVE
2 brioche buns
50g bistro salad
½ cucumber, thinly sliced with
    a Y-peeler

A smoky, flavoursome burger with all the colours and textures. So quick to rustle up, yet satisfying, this is perfect for either lunch or a light dinner. We normally serve this with extra salad and grated carrot, or whatever salad ingredients we have left in the fridge.

1. Preheat the oven to 180°C/160°C fan/gas 4 and line a baking tray with parchment paper.

2. Rub the Chinese five spice over the duck breasts, place on the lined baking tray and bake for 20 minutes until cooked through.

3. Remove the duck breasts from the oven and rest on a plate for 15 minutes to cool then discard the skin and shred the meat using two forks.

4. Coat the base of a frying pan with spray light oil and fry the carrot, spring onions and red onion for 5 minutes over a medium heat. Add the shredded duck and stir together along with the soy and hoisin sauces.

5. Slice the brioche buns in half and place a bed of bistro salad on the bottom of each bun. Pile on the shredded duck and top with the sliced cucumber and bun lid.

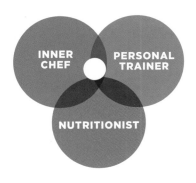

INNER CHEF
PERSONAL TRAINER
NUTRITIONIST

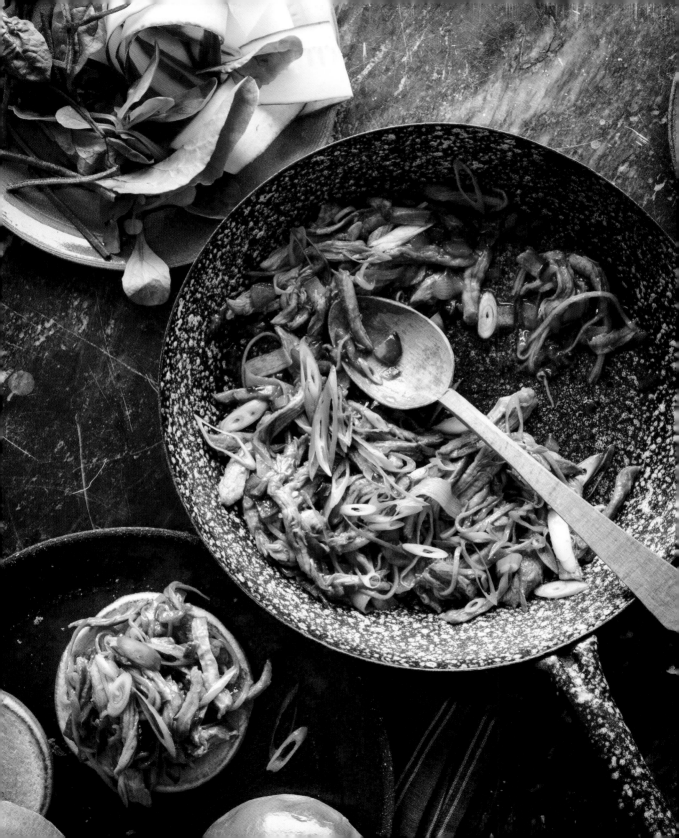

CALORIES 505
PROTEIN 30g
FAT 26g
CARBS 38g
SUGARS 8g

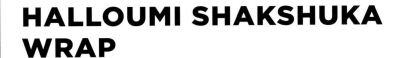

HALLOUMI SHAKSHUKA WRAP

SERVES 1

Preparation time: 5 minutes
Cooking time: 10 minutes

2 tbsp tomato purée
1 wholemeal tortilla wrap
50g avocado
1 egg
60g halloumi, sliced
20g baby spinach leaves
sea salt and freshly ground
    black pepper
spray light oil for frying

Easy and filling, this is equally good for both lunch or breakfast. A vegetarian option, loaded with protein to keep you full until your next feed! Halloumi is one of my favourite cheeses so I had to put this one in here.

1. Spread the tomato purée on the tortilla wrap leaving a 2-cm border around the edge.

2. Mash the avocado onto the tomato purée and season with salt and pepper.

3. In a small frying pan, fry the egg in a thin coating of spray light oil over a medium-high heat until cooked to your liking.

4. Place the fried egg on top of the avocado mash then fry the halloumi for 2 minutes on each side in the same pan, until golden on each side.

5. Place the halloumi slices on top of the fried egg, add the spinach and fold the wrap. Cut in half and serve.

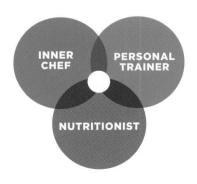

INNER CHEF
PERSONAL TRAINER
NUTRITIONIST

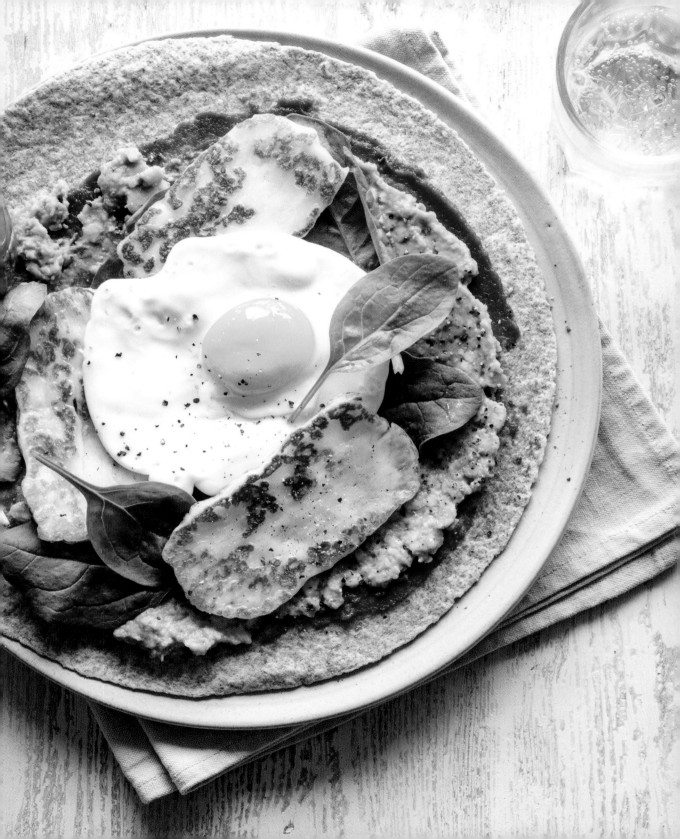

CALORIES 362
PROTEIN 47g
FAT 11g
CARBS 16g
SUGARS 11g

NICOISE SALAD

Preparation time: 5 minutes
Cooking time: 10 minutes

100g Tenderstem broccoli
½ red onion, thinly sliced
90g cherry tomatoes
80g fine green beans
1 egg
120g can tuna in water, drained
15g pitted black olives
freshly ground black pepper
spray light oil for cooking

FOR THE DRESSING
1 tbsp Dijon mustard
½ tbsp red wine vinegar
1 tbsp apple cider vinegar

So simple to make and easy to eat, both in summer and winter.
There are lots of textures, tastes and colours going on, which
makes you appreciate this dish for more than just its simplicity!

1. Start by making the dressing in a small bowl. Mix together the
   Dijon mustard, red wine vinegar and apple cider vinegar and
   set aside.

2. Spray the base of a frying pan with spray light oil, add the
   Tenderstem broccoli, onion, tomatoes and green beans and fry
   over a medium heat for 10 minutes until the green beans and
   broccoli are just tender.

3. Meanwhile, boil the egg in a small saucepan for 7 minutes, then
   run under cold water to stop it cooking any further.

4. Place the vegetables in a pasta bowl and top with the tuna
   and black olives. Peel the egg, slice it in half and place on top.
   Season everything with a little black pepper and finally drizzle
   the Dijon mustard dressing on top.

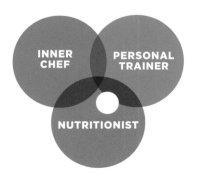

INNER
CHEF

PERSONAL
TRAINER

NUTRITIONIST

CALORIES 649
PROTEIN 53g
FAT 18g
CARBS 69g
SUGARS 12g

**SERVES
1–2**

ULTIMATE TUNA MELT

Preparation time: 5 minutes
Cooking time: 10 minutes

120g can tuna in water, drained
65g Lighter than Light
   mayonnaise
1 tbsp lemon juice
2 spring onions, chopped
25g spinach leaves
2 large slices sourdough bread
1 tomato, sliced
30g Red Leicester cheese,
   grated
sea salt and freshly ground
   black pepper
spray light oil for cooking

Yes, this is a calorific sandwich, BUT it's also packed with nutrient-dense calories. It's all about choosing to eat the right meal at the right time for whatever your goal is.

1. In a small mixing bowl, mix together the tuna, mayonnaise, lemon juice and spring onions along with a pinch each of salt and pepper.

2. Place the spinach leaves on one of the slices of bread, followed by the tuna mayo. Place the slices of tomato over the top of the tuna then sprinkle over the cheese to finish. Top with the second slice of sourdough to complete the sandwich.

3. Coat the base of a frying pan with spray light oil and place over a medium heat. Also lightly spray the side of the sandwich you are going to lay in the pan first.

4. Cook the sandwich for 2–3 minutes and carefully check to see if the bread has turned golden on the bottom. Spray the top side of the sandwich with the oil and flip over for the other half to cook, again for 2–3 minutes.

5. Note: this is quite a big sandwich and could be shared between two people with a simple green salad.

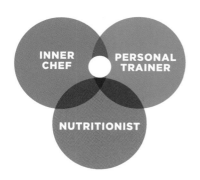

INNER
CHEF

PERSONAL
TRAINER

NUTRITIONIST

**CALORIES 420
PROTEIN 54g
FAT 9g
CARBS 17g
SUGARS 11g**

LOW-CARB CHICKEN & BACON PESTO NOODLES

SERVES 2

Preparation time: 5 minutes
Cooking time: 25 minutes

1 white onion, finely chopped
2 skinless chicken breasts, chopped into chunks
2 smoked bacon medallions, finely sliced
1 green pepper, sliced
100g frozen peas
100g frozen fine green beans
1 chicken stock cube
20g green pesto
250g packet of shirataki noodles
100g Philadelphia Lightest cream cheese (or other low-fat cream cheese)
10g pine nuts
20g Parmesan, grated
spray light olive oil for cooking

You'll struggle to find another recipe that packs as much protein and flavour into a single bowl. Really easy to make, we enjoy twisting the smoky bacon and cheese-flavoured noodles with chunks of juicy chicken and crunchy pine nuts that are wrapped in between.

1. Lightly coat the base of a large frying pan with spray light oil and place over a medium heat. Add the onion, chicken and bacon to the pan and cook, stirring, until cooked through. This should take 8–10 minutes. Add the green pepper, peas and green beans and cook for a further 5 minutes.

2. Add 100ml of boiling water to the pan and crumble in the chicken stock cube, then add the pesto and stir everything together. Reduce the heat and simmer for 2–3 minutes.

3. Add the noodles, stir everything together well and cook for a further 3–4 minutes to ensure the noodles are hot. Add the cream cheese and stir until everything is coated in the creamy pesto sauce.

4. Divide between two warmed pasta bowls and sprinkle the pine nuts and Parmesan on top.

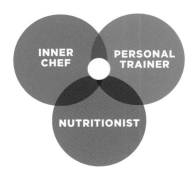

INNER CHEF
PERSONAL TRAINER
NUTRITIONIST

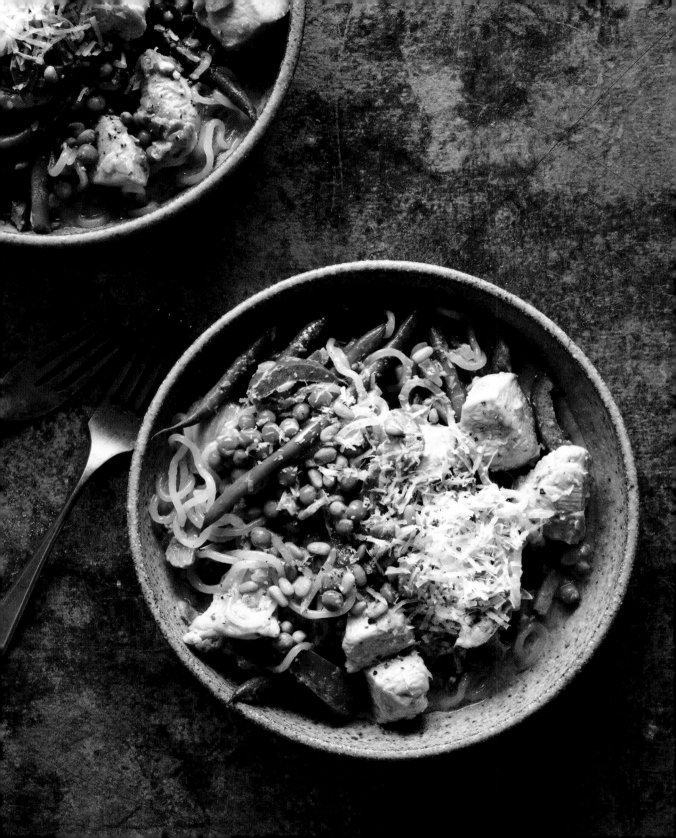

CALORIES 451
PROTEIN 21g
FAT 10g
CARBS 35g
SUGARS 15g

SERVES 4

THAI FISHCAKES WITH MANGO & CHILLI DRESSING

Preparation time: 30 minutes
Cooking time: 45 minutes

500g salmon fillet
600g sweet potato, peeled and
    chopped
4 spring onions, finely chopped
40g green Thai curry paste
1 tbsp lemongrass paste
1 tbsp light soy sauce
3 tbsp lime juice
30g fresh coriander, finely
    chopped
1 green chilli, deseeded and finely
    chopped
sea salt and freshly ground black
    pepper
spray light oil for cooking

FOR THE THAI GREEN SALAD
1 tbsp green Thai curry paste
1 tbsp lime juice
2 tsp sesame oil
160g gem lettuce, shredded
100g spinach leaves
1 red onion, finely sliced
500g cucumber, diced

FOR THE MANGO & CHILLI DRESSING
150g fresh mango, peeled and
    diced
7 tbsp water
2 tsp chilli purée
2 tsp apple cider vinegar

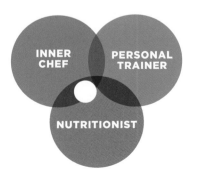

Our Thai fishcake recipe is fresh, zesty and with just the right amount of spice to give each serving a little 'kick' with our homemade mango and chilli dressing. Although preparing these can take a little longer than other recipes in this book, they're ideal for anyone looking for high-protein, low-carb meal prep ideas that they can make at the weekend then eat throughout the week.

1. Preheat the oven to 200°C/180°C fan/gas 6.

2. Season the salmon with a good pinch each of salt and pepper and wrap in aluminium foil. Place on a baking tray and cook in the oven for 15 minutes. When the salmon is cooked, remove it from the oven, unwrap it and set aside to cool.

3. Place the sweet potato in another baking tin, coat with spray light oil and bake in the oven for 30 minutes. Remove and set aside to cool for 15 minutes then mash until smooth.

4. While the salmon and sweet potato are cooking, blend together all the ingredients for the mango chilli dressing (adding a splash more water if it needs thinning a little) and set aside.

5. In a large mixing bowl, mix together the spring onions, curry paste, lemongrass paste, soy sauce, lime juice, coriander and green chilli. Stir through the mashed sweet potato and flake in the salmon, discarding the skin.

6. Use a fork to mix everything together until evenly combined then, with clean hands, mould the fishcake mix into 12 patties. Be careful while doing this as the fishcakes will be quite delicate.

7. To make the salad, mix the curry paste, lime juice and sesame oil together in a bowl then add the remainder of the salad ingredients and toss together before seasoning, to taste.

8. Heat a large frying pan over low-medium heat and cover the base with spray light oil. Place the patties in the pan and cook for 3–4 minutes on each side, being very careful when you turn them so they don't break apart.

9. Serve three fishcakes per person along with the salad and finish with a good drizzle of the mango dressing.

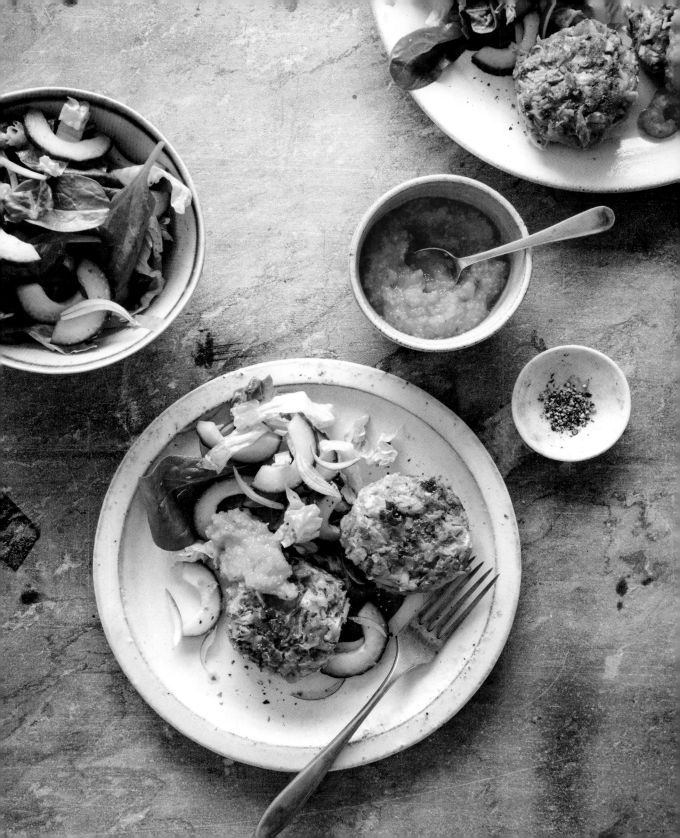

Dinner

This section has been inspired by some of my favourite recipes from around the world, including the very best of Middle Eastern and West Asian cuisine. There's also the greatest barbecue recipe you'll ever see (bold statement, I know) and healthy 'fakeaway' alternatives. All so your taste buds are never bored, but your dietary goals are always supported.

CALORIES 735
PROTEIN 49g
FAT 35g
CARBS 53g
SUGARS 12g

SERVES
2

NANDO'S FAKE AWAY

Preparation time: 20 minutes +
     marinating
Cooking time: 20 minutes

1 whole chicken
2 corn on the cob
2 wholemeal pita breads

FOR THE MARINADE
juice of 1 lemon
1 tsp dried parsley
1 tsp dried rosemary
1 tsp dried coriander
¼ tsp turmeric
½ tsp garlic purée
1 tsp apple cider vinegar

FOR THE GUACAMOLE DIP
100g avocado
½ red onion, finely diced
juice of ½ lime

FOR THE SALSA
80g cherry tomatoes, halved
juice of ½ lime
½ tsp chilli salsa purée
1 red pepper, finely diced

FOR THE FETA & SUN-DRIED
     TOMATO SALAD
large handful of spinach
60g feta cheese, diced
30g sun-dried tomatoes,
     chopped
100g cucumber, finely diced
juice of ½ lemon

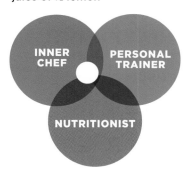

A healthier take on a dish from everyone's favourite go-to
restaurant that's ideal on a hot summer's day. What's better
than a stuffed chicken pita, served with a fresh feta and sun-
dried tomato salad, that's high in protein and healthy fats and
seasoned to perfection?

1. Place all the marinade ingredients in a small mixing bowl and
   mix together well. Coat the chicken in the marinade, place it
   on a baking tray, then cover with tin foil and leave to marinate
   in the fridge for a minimum of 4 hours, ideally overnight.

2. Preheat the oven to 190°C/170°C fan/gas 5 and take the
   chicken out of the fridge 30 minutes before you start cooking.

3. Place the chicken in the oven and cook it for 45 minutes per
   kilo plus 20 minutes. So, a 1.4kg chicken will take 1 hour 25
   minutes. Remove the foil for the final 10 minutes of cooking.
   Leave to rest for 20 minutes before carving. The chicken will
   serve 5 people, so you'll have plenty of leftovers for meals
   through the week.

4. While the chicken is cooking, make the guacamole by mashing
   the avocado together with the red onion and lime juice and
   season to taste.

5. To make the salsa, simply mix all the salsa ingredients together
   in a small bowl.

6. To make the feta and sun-dried tomato salad, again, simply
   mix all the salad ingredients together in a bowl.

7. Boil the corn on the cobs for 10 minutes and finally, just before
   you serve, pop the pita breads in a toaster so they are nice
   and warm. To serve, stuff the chicken and sides into the pita
   breads and serve the corn cob on the side.

Tip: If you prefer, you could marinate 2 chicken breasts and cook
them in the oven for 20 minutes, removing the foil for the final 5
minutes of cooking.

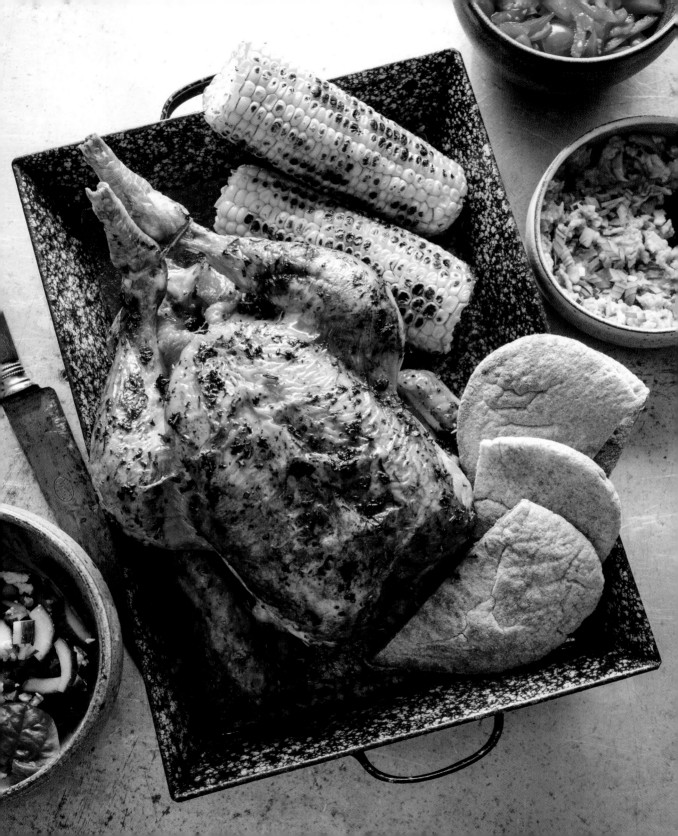

CALORIES 630
PROTEIN 35g
FAT 22g
CARBS 74g
SUGARS 30g

SERVES 2

Preparation time: 10 minutes
Cooking time: 15 minutes

1 red onion, finely chopped
3 spring onions, finely chopped
225g rump beef steak, thinly sliced
100g baby peppers, finely sliced
50g spring green cabbage, shredded
100g sugar snap peas
6 bao buns
white sesame seeds, for sprinkling
spray light oil for cooking

FOR THE STICKY HONEY SAUCE
1 tbsp honey
3 tbsp light soy sauce
½ tsp garlic purée

STICKY BEEF BAO BUNS

If you're looking for new ways to meet your protein requirements for the day then look no further. Presenting a batch of soft, sticky, steamed bao buns. Possibly the greatest culinary creation from China, each one is packed with flavour and the individual servings make portion control that much easier.

1. Coat the base of a large frying pan with spray light oil and fry the red onion, spring onions and steak over a medium-high heat for a few minutes. Add the remainder of the vegetables and let them soften slightly and add a generous pinch of black pepper.

2. In small bowl, make the sauce by mixing the honey, soy sauce and garlic purée together. Add to the beef stir-fry and bring to a slight boil to let the sauce thicken. This should only take a couple of minutes. Then turn off the heat.

3. Microwave the bao buns according to the pack instructions (or if you like them a little crispy, like we do, place the bao buns on a baking tray in an oven preheated to 180°C/160°C fan/gas 4 for 4–5 minutes.)

4. To serve, stuff the bao buns with the sticky beef stir-fry and sprinkle over some sesame seeds. Then ... enjoy!

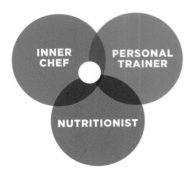

INNER CHEF **PERSONAL TRAINER** **NUTRITIONIST**

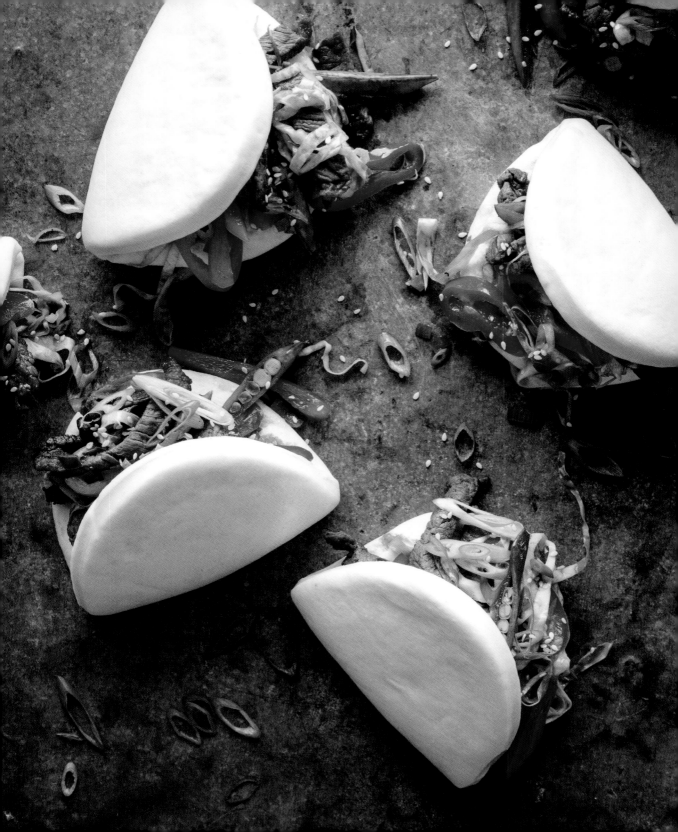

SERVES 2

DUCK DONBURI

Preparation time: 5 minutes
Cooking time: 35 minutes

2 duck breast fillets
1 red onion, finely chopped
1 carrot, peeled into long thin strips
80g mangetout
50g edamame beans, fresh or frozen
2 eggs
250g packet of pre-cooked basmati rice
spray light oil for cooking

FOR THE SWEET TERIYAKI SAUCE
1 tsp ginger purée
½ tsp garlic purée
2 tbsp honey
1 tsp arrowroot, mixed with 1 tbsp water
3 tbsp light soy sauce

TO GARNISH
¼ cucumber, cut into long thin strips
2 spring onions, sliced
sesame seeds, for sprinkling

Duck donburi is a Japanese take on a duck teriyaki rice bowl. Oven-baked duck breast fillets, shredded and coated in a sweet honey teriyaki sauce and mixed with crunchy stir-fried vegetables. It's served over a bowl of white rice and is ideal for anyone wanting to mix up their protein intake, as it delivers a new amino acid profile to your muscles and fresh tastes and textures to your taste buds.

1. Preheat the oven to 190°C/170°C fan/gas 5 and line a baking tray with parchment paper.

2. Place the duck breasts on the lined baking tray and bake for 20 minutes until cooked through.

3. Remove the duck breasts from the oven and rest on a plate for 15 minutes to cool then discard the skin and shred the meat using two forks. Cover with aluminium foil and set aside while you prepare the sauce.

4. Coat the base of a frying pan with spray light oil, set over a medium heat and sauté the red onion until starting to soften. Add the carrot, mangetout and edamame beans and stir until cooked. This should only take around 5–7 minutes as you want to make sure the vegetables still have some crunch.

5. While the vegetables are cooking, add all of the sauce ingredients to a small saucepan over a low heat. Turn up the heat to medium and stir regularly until the sauce comes to a simmer and thickens slightly, then immediately take off the heat.

6. Place the shredded duck in the teriyaki sauce and stir to coat the duck with the sticky sauce.

7. To fry the eggs, set a non-stick or ceramic pan with a lid over a medium heat. Coat the base of the pan with spray light oil and allow it to get hot before cracking the eggs into the pan. Place the lid on the pan and cook for a couple of minutes or to the way you like your eggs.

8. Heat the packet of pre-cooked rice according to the pack instructions and divide between two warmed bowls before spooning the stir-fried vegetables and duck teriyaki over the rice. Finish the dish with the cucumber, spring onions and sesame seeds and top with the fried eggs.

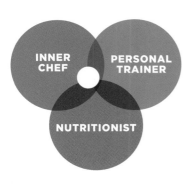

INNER CHEF
PERSONAL TRAINER
NUTRITIONIST

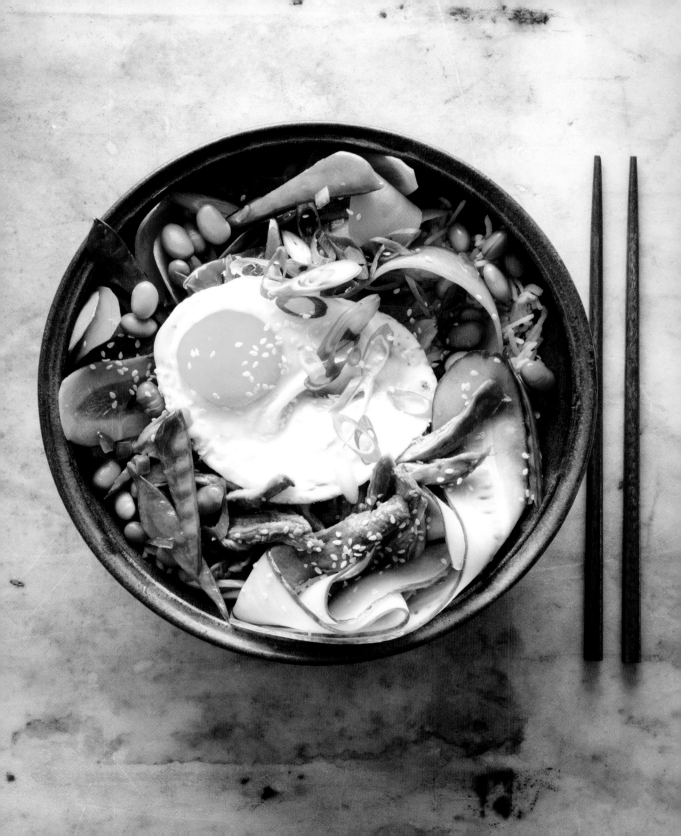

SATAY CHICKEN

SERVES 2

Preparation time: 15 minutes +
5 hours marinating
Cooking time: 25 minutes

500g skinless chicken breasts,
sliced into long, thin strips

FOR THE SATAY SAUCE MARINADE
80g peanut butter, smooth or
crunchy
80g 0%-fat yogurt
1 tbsp light soy sauce
1 tbsp clear honey
2 tsp curry powder
1 tsp ginger purée
½ tsp garlic purée
1 tsp red chilli paste
spray light oil for cooking

FOR THE STIR-FRY
80g beansprouts
100g Tenderstem broccoli,
roughly chopped
100g white cabbage, shredded
3 spring onions, roughly
chopped
50g carrots, cut into thin
matchsticks
1 tbsp light soy sauce
15g roasted peanuts, roughly
chopped
100g cucumber, thinly sliced
½ lime, cut into wedges
10g/⅓ bunch fresh coriander

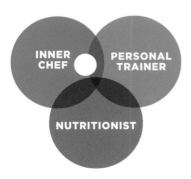

Locked and loaded chicken satay skewers! Naturally packed with protein and healthy fats to which we have included a larger amount of chicken, so the skewers are full. I don't know about anyone else but my heart sinks when a kebab skewer is sparse and more skewer is on show than meat! Marinated for over 5 hours then cooked until juicy and tender with a thick layer of satay sauce bubbling away and a little extra to drizzle over the top. If you are counting calories you don't have to have as big a portion as the recipe states – quantities in the recipe can simply be halved.

1. In a large mixing bowl, whisk together all the marinade ingredients and set aside 2 tablespoons of the mix for drizzling over the finished dish. Add the chicken to the marinade and spoon the marinade over the meat, making sure the sauce fully coats the chicken. Cover the bowl and leave in the fridge for 5 hours to marinate.

2. Preheat the oven to 200°C/180°C fan/gas 6, line a baking tray with parchment paper and soak four wooden skewers in a bowl of cold water for 5 minutes.

3. Pat the skewers dry with kitchen towel, thread the chicken onto the skewers and place them on the lined baking tray. (I like to use a deep tray and rest the ends of the skewers on the edge of the tray so the chicken isn't touching the bottom so that the fat drains away easier.) Pour the remainder of the marinade over the chicken skewers and place them in the oven for 20 minutes, turning halfway through the cooking time, until the chicken is cooked and the marinade has caught a little.

4. When the chicken is nearly done, lightly coat the base of a wok or frying pan with spray light oil and fry the beansprouts, Tenderstem, cabbage, spring onions and carrots over a medium heat for 5 minutes before adding the soy sauce.

5. To serve, place the stir-fried vegetables in pasta bowls and add the chicken by using a fork to slide it off the skewers. Pour over the reserved satay sauce (it may need thinning out a little, if so, add a splash of almond milk and give it a good stir). Finally, decorate with a sprinkle of roasted peanuts, some cucumber slices, a couple of lime wedges and a scattering of coriander.

CALORIES 699
PROTEIN 48g
FAT 46g
CARBS 19g
SUGARS 8g

SERVES 4

CHILLI CON CARNE MEATBALLS

Preparation time: 30 minutes
Cooking time: 35 minutes

FOR THE MEATBALLS
750g beef and pork mince
1 tsp chilli powder
1 tsp smoked paprika
1 egg
sea salt and freshly ground
    black pepper
spray light oil for cooking

FOR THE CHILLI CON CARNE SAUCE
1 red pepper, roughly chopped
1 green pepper, roughly
    chopped
½ courgette, roughly chopped
1 red onion, chopped
400g tin mixed beans, drained
½ tsp garlic purée
400g tin chopped tomatoes
1 tsp ginger purée
1 tsp chilli pepper purée
200ml beef stock

TO SERVE
250g fresh green beans or
    Tenderstem or broccoli,
    trimmed

This has become one of my favourite recipes to have on a British winter evening. Flavour-packed pork and beef meatballs simmering in a sweet tomato sauce, these can also be accompanied with a large serving of rice if you need to 'carb up' before a big training session.

1. To prepare the meatballs, place the mince, chilli powder, smoked paprika and egg along with a good pinch each of salt and pepper into a mixing bowl. Use your hands to mix everything together and roll into 16 golf ball-sized balls.

2. Heat a large frying pan over a medium heat, coat the base of the pan with spray light oil and place the meatballs in the pan to cook. Use tongs to turn the meatballs, making sure they are cooked on every side with a crispy edge. This should take about 10 minutes. At this point a lot of fat will come out of the meat, drain this off onto kitchen towel and discard.

3. Place the red and green peppers, courgette and onion into the frying pan with the meatballs and sauté for 5 minutes until the vegetables have softened a little.

4. Add the remaining ingredients to the frying pan and bring to the boil. Immediately turn down the heat to low and let the chilli simmer for 20 minutes.

5. Meanwhile, cook the green beans and Tenderstem or broccoli in salted water for 5–6 minutes until they have just a bit of bite left then drain. Serve alongside the chilli.

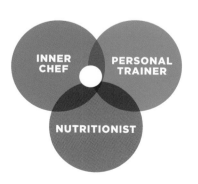

INNER CHEF

PERSONAL TRAINER

NUTRITIONIST

SERVES 2

CHEESEBURGER PIZZA

Preparation time: 45 minutes +
30 minutes proving
Cooking time: 20 minutes

FOR ENOUGH DOUGH FOR 4
PIZZAS (SPARE DOUGH CAN BE
FROZEN)
3 tsp zero-calorie granulated
white sugar replacer
1½ tsp active dry yeast
500g strong white bread flour

FOR THE CHEESEBURGER
TOPPING (PER PIZZA)
125g lean minced beef
80g passata
25g reduced-sugar tomato
ketchup
25g pickled gherkins, sliced
20g Red Leicester cheese,
grated
30g 50% less fat Cheddar
cheese, grated
½ red onion, thinly sliced

FOR THE BURGER SAUCE
1 shallot, finely chopped
200g pickled gherkins
¼ tsp mustard powder
½ tsp ground paprika
½ tsp tomato purée
½ tsp onion powder

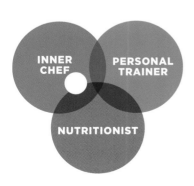

The reason I love this recipe is because it's a hybrid of a cheeseburger and a pizza. Combining the best of both worlds, it's great to share or just devour on your own if you need a carb boost before training. Finally, the real secret weapon of this particular culinary creation is the burger sauce, which is a healthier, low-calorie version of even the best fast-food takeaways. See photo on the next page.

1. In a small bowl, mix 1 teaspoon of the sweetener and the active dry yeast together with 100ml of warm water and set aside for 10 minutes for the yeast to activate. After 10 minutes the mixture should smell very yeasty with bubbles floating to the surface. (It is important to use warm water, if the water is too hot it can kill the yeast, if it is too cold the yeast will not activate.)

2. Using a stand mixer or a large bowl and wooden spoon, mix together 180ml of hot water and the remaining sweetener. Leave to cool slightly then add 400g of the bread flour and mix well.

3. Add the yeast mix along with the remaining bread flour. If you have a stand mixer, beat the dough with a dough hook for 5 minutes, then take the dough out of the bowl, place on a lightly floured work surface and knead by hand a few times, forming the dough into a ball. If you don't have a stand mixer knead the dough by hand for around 10 minutes until the dough is nice and smooth.

4. Return the kneaded dough to the mixing bowl, cover with a clean tea towel and leave in a warm place for 30 minutes to prove. It should double in size.

5. Meanwhile, prepare the toppings. Lightly coat the base of a small frying pan with spray light oil and cook the beef mince over a medium heat until browned. In a small bowl, mix the passata and tomato ketchup together.

6. To make the burger sauce, lightly fry the shallot in a little spray light oil until soft, then place in a blender with the remaining sauce ingredients and blitz together until smooth.

¼ tsp garlic powder
1 tbsp wholegrain mustard
1 tsp turmeric
2 tbsp mirin
2 tbsp gherkin water
3 tbsp Lighter than Light
  mayonnaise

7. When the dough has doubled in size, heat the oven to its hottest temperature (this is usually about 220–250°C) and place a baking sheet in the oven to heat up.

8. Divide the dough into four balls and roll each one out on a lightly floured work surface. You want each pizza base quite thin, about 5mm, and an even thickness all over.

9. Spread the tomato sauce over the base, leaving a 1-cm border round the edge, then scatter over the cooked mince followed by the remaining toppings. Drizzle over a little of the burger sauce before carefully sliding your pizza onto the preheated baking tray.

10. Cook for 8–9 minutes until the crust is golden and the cheese is bubbling. Drizzle with a little more sauce and tuck in!

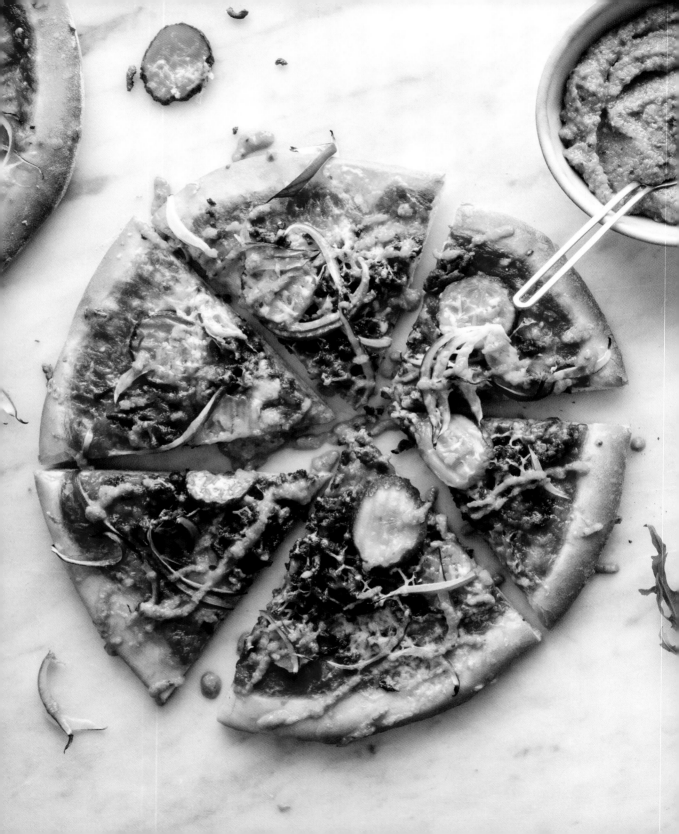

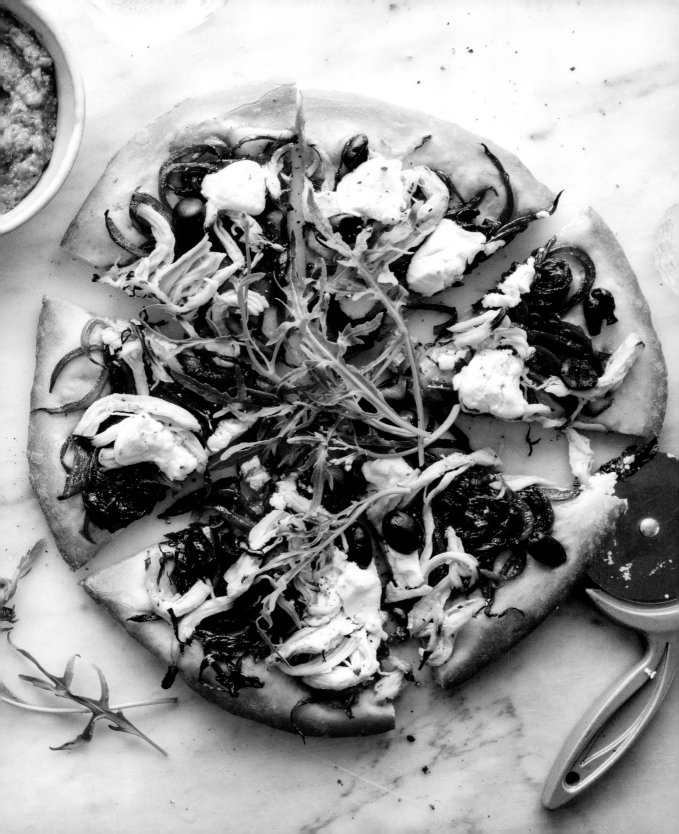

CALORIES 503
PROTEIN 33g
FAT 13g
CARBS 76g
SUGARS 16g

SERVES 2

CARAMELISED ONION, HONEY CHICKEN & GOATS' CHEESE PIZZA

Preparation time: 30 minutes + proving
Cooking time: 20 minutes

FOR ENOUGH DOUGH FOR 4 PIZZAS (SPARE DOUGH CAN BE FROZEN)
3 tsp zero-calorie granulated white sugar replacer
1½ tsp active dry yeast
500g strong white bread flour

FOR THE TOPPING (PER PIZZA)
1 skinless chicken breast
1 tbsp clear honey
2 red onions, thinly sliced
2 tbsp zero-calorie granulated white sugar replacer
4 tbsp balsamic vinegar
70g soft goats' cheese
30g black pitted olives, halved
handful of rocket leaves
spray light oil for cooking

This is our take on a more sophisticated pizza. Sweet and juicy caramelised onions melting into a thin and crispy base, topped with honey-glazed shredded chicken and rocket salad. It tastes absolutely immense! I think we also have to mention, the dimensions of the pizza below serve two people, as half a pizza equates in size to one medium-sized pizza. So don't worry if you're sharing with someone with a massive appetite, because there's plenty for the pair of you, or for leftovers for the next day. See photo on the previous page.

1. Start making the dough by mixing 1 teaspoon of the sweetener and the active dry yeast together with 100ml of warm water in a small bowl and set aside for 10 minutes for the yeast to activate. After 10 minutes the mixture should be frothy and bubbly and smell very yeasty. (It is important to use warm water; if the water is too hot it can kill the yeast, if it is too cold the yeast will not activate.)

2. Using a stand mixer or a large bowl and wooden spoon, mix together 180ml of hot water and the remaining sweetener. Leave to cool slightly then add 400g of the bread flour and mix well.

3. Add the yeast mix along with the remaining bread flour. If you have a stand mixer, beat the dough with a dough hook for 5 minutes, then take the dough out of the bowl and knead it by hand a few times, shaping it into a ball. If you don't have a stand mixer, knead with your hands for around 10 minutes until the dough is nice and smooth.

4. Place the kneaded dough back in the mixing bowl, cover with a clean tea towel and leave in a warm place for 30 minutes, until doubled in size.

5. Meanwhile, preheat the oven to its hottest temperature (usually about 220–250°C) and place a flat baking sheet in the oven to heat up too.

6. Bring a small saucepan of water to the boil and poach the chicken breast for 10 minutes until cooked through. Remove the chicken from the pan, shred with two forks and toss the honey through the shredded chicken.

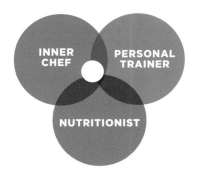

INNER CHEF
PERSONAL TRAINER
NUTRITIONIST

7. Coat the base of a frying pan with spray light oil and fry the red onions over a medium heat until soft, then add the sweetener and balsamic vinegar. The onions should become dark and sticky. Set the onions aside.

8. After the dough has doubled in size, divide it into four balls. On a floured work surface, roll out one of the dough balls to about 4mm thick.

9. Cover the pizza base with the caramelised onions. This is the equivalent of a tomato base, so ensure all the base is covered evenly. Scatter over the honey chicken, crumble over the goats' cheese and finally drop the olives on top.

10. Carefully slide the pizza onto the preheated baking sheet and cook for 8–9 minutes until the crust is golden and the chicken is just starting to colour.

11. Take the pizza out of the oven and top with the rocket leaves.

CALORIES 692
PROTEIN 239g
FAT 19g
CARBS 32g
SUGARS 37g

**SERVES
6**

CHILLI BEEF NACHOS

Preparation time: 20 minutes
Cooking time: 40–50 minutes

240g lightly salted nachos
100g 50% reduced-fat Cheddar
   cheese, grated
300g guacamole (see page 102)

FOR THE CHILLI
2 red onions, diced
1kg lean beef mince, less than
   5% fat
1 tsp smoked paprika
1 tsp chilli powder
1 red pepper, sliced
1 green pepper, sliced
200g frozen peas
200g green beans
400g tin chopped tomatoes
½ tsp garlic purée
1 tsp chilli purée
400g tin mixed beans, drained
sea salt and freshly ground
   black pepper
spray light oil for cooking

This recipe makes a strong case for being the best high-protein dish for a chilled movie night. There's no better feeling than getting into your dressing gown and slippers, putting your feet up and dipping a warm crispy nacho into the smoky chilli dip and fresh, creamy guacamole!

1. Coat the base of a large saucepan with some spray light oil and sauté the onions on a medium heat for 10 minutes until they are soft. Add the beef mince and break it up while stirring in the smoked paprika, chilli powder and a good pinch each of salt and pepper. Once the meat has browned add the peppers, peas and green beans.

2. Add the chopped tomatoes, garlic purée and chilli purée along with the mixed beans.

3. Bring the chilli to the boil then turn down the heat to a slow simmer, stirring now and then to make sure nothing sticks to the bottom of the pan. Cook for 30 minutes, or a little longer if you want a thicker consistency.

4. Preheat the oven to 200°C/180°C fan/gas 6 then place the nachos in the oven 5 minutes before serving to warm up.

5. Serve the hot chilli on top of the crispy nachos and sprinkle over the grated cheese.

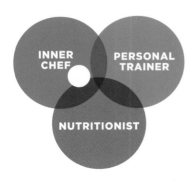

INNER
CHEF

PERSONAL
TRAINER

NUTRITIONIST

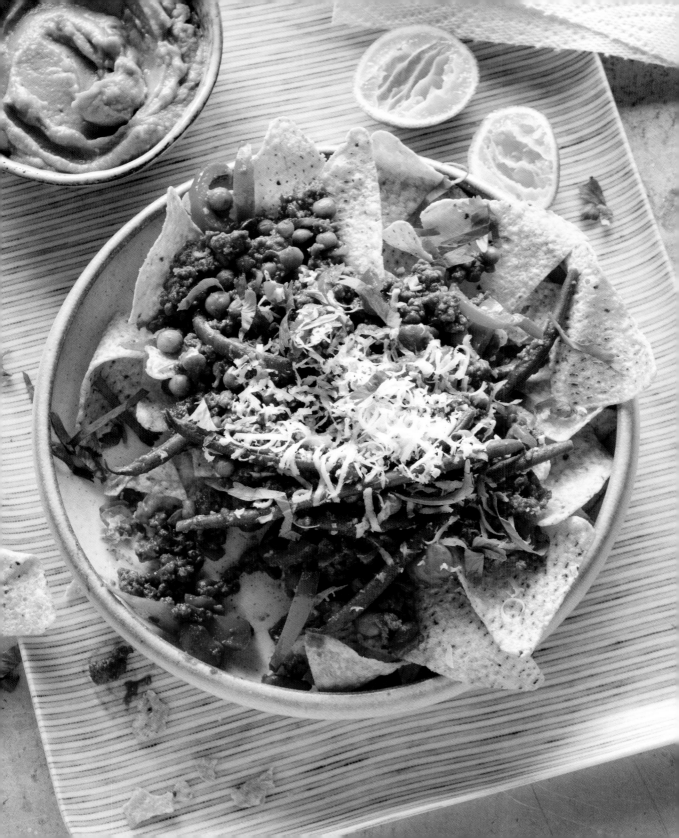

CALORIES 429
PROTEIN 17g
FAT 14g
CARBS 26g
SUGARS 19g

SALMON CHILLI TERIYAKI SHIRATAKI NOODLE BOWL

Preparation time: 10 minutes
Cooking time: 20 minutes

2 salmon fillets
juice of ½ lemon
½ courgette, roughly chopped
1 red pepper, sliced
50g edamame beans
3 spring onions, finely chopped
1 red onion, sliced
250g shirataki noodles
1 tbsp light soy sauce
sea salt and freshly ground
    black pepper
spray light oil for cooking

FOR THE CHILLI TERIYAKI SAUCE
1 tsp ginger purée
½ tsp garlic purée
1 tbsp honey
2 tsp dried chilli flakes
3 tbsp light soy sauce

Shirataki noodles (also known as konjac noodles, since they come from the root of the konjac plant) can be a powerful tool in your arsenal if you're looking to lower your calorie intake for the day. This is because they're high in glucomannan, a type of fibre that (in some studies) has been shown to help suppress appetite. They have very little flavour of their own, but are so versatile and can absorb and take on the flavours of the dish you're pairing them with. Our kitchen is rarely without several packs of shirataki noodles.

1. Preheat the oven to 180°C/160°C fan/gas 4.

2. Wrap the salmon fillets in an aluminium foil parcel with a squeeze of lemon juice and a pinch each of salt and pepper. Bake in the oven for 15–20 minutes, until the fillets flake when gently pressed.

3. Place the chilli teriyaki sauce ingredients in a small saucepan and cook over a low heat until thickened slightly.

4. When the salmon has been in the oven for 10 minutes, coat the base of a large frying pan with spray light oil and fry the vegetables over a medium-high heat for 5 minutes until they have softened slightly but still retain some crunch. Add the noodles and soy sauce and cook for a few minutes more, until the noodles are hot.

5. Serve the vegetable noodle stir-fry in pasta bowls and place the salmon fillet on top. Pour the sticky teriyaki sauce over to finish.

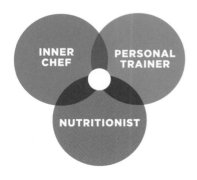

INNER CHEF

PERSONAL TRAINER

NUTRITIONIST

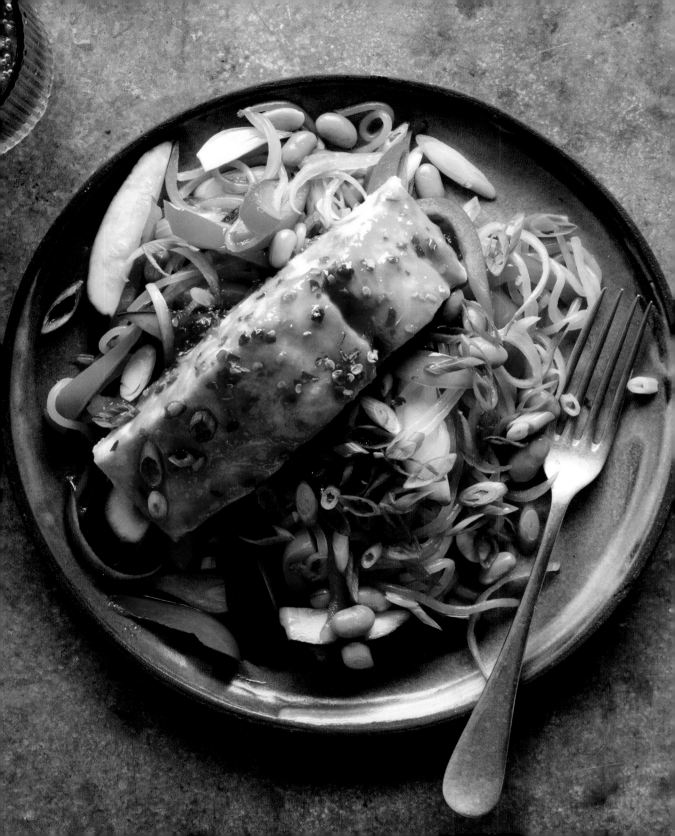

CALORIES 526
PROTEIN 41g
FAT 9g
CARBS 111g
SUGARS 26g

SWEET & TANGY PORK

Preparation time: 10 minutes
Cooking time: 20 minutes

2 pork chops, cut into thin
    slices
1 red onion, thinly sliced
1 yellow pepper, cut into 2-cm
    chunks
1 red pepper, cut into 2-cm
    chunks
3 spring onions, roughly
    chopped
100g baby corn, chopped into
    small chunks
spray light oil for cooking

FOR THE SWEET AND SOUR SAUCE
½ x 430g tin of pineapple
    chunks in juice
100ml passata
2 tbsp rice vinegar
1 tbsp zero-calorie granulated
    white sugar replacer
1 tbsp light soy sauce

FOR THE EGG-FRIED RICE
250g packet of pre-cooked
    long grain rice
½ white onion, finely chopped
1 egg, beaten

This recipe is perfect when you're needing something new to mix up your protein intake. A fresh, clean take on sweet and sour, you combine a selection of nutrient-dense vegetables with lean cuts of crispy pork, then cover it with a low-calorie sweet and tangy sauce.

1. Coat the base of a large frying pan with spray light oil and place over a medium heat. Cook the pork slices in the pan along with the red onion for 5 minutes, until the onion is soft and starting to turn brown at the edges. Add the peppers, spring onions and baby corn and cook for about 10 minutes, until the vegetables have started to soften but still retain some crunch.

2. Meanwhile, place the sweet and sour sauce ingredients in a small bowl and mix together. Pour the sauce into the pan and bring to a simmer over a medium heat to thicken it slightly. This should take about 7–10 minutes.

3. To prepare the egg-fried rice, microwave the packet of pre-cooked rice according to the pack instructions. While the rice is heating up, coat the base of a frying pan with spray light oil and lightly fry the onion. Add the hot rice to the frying pan and mix with the fried onion, then push to one side of the pan. Add the beaten egg to the empty side of the pan and gently scramble before mixing through the rice and onion.

4. Divide the rice between two warmed plates and spoon the sweet and sour pork over the rice, to serve.

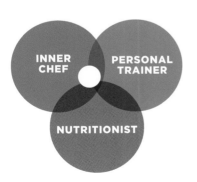

CALORIES 673
PROTEIN 56g
FAT 27g
CARBS 47g
SUGARS 31g

SERVES
2

CHICKEN PAD THAI

Preparation time: 10 minutes
Cooking time: 15 minutes

100g dried rice noodles
2 skinless chicken breasts, cut
  into thin strips
3 spring onions, chopped
150g beansprouts
2 eggs, beaten
15g roasted peanuts, roughly
  chopped
½ lime, cut into 2 wedges
spray light oil for cooking

FOR THE SAUCE
1 white shallot
3 tbsp tamarind paste
2 tbsp dark brown sugar
½ tbsp fish sauce
1 tsp light soy sauce
6 tbsp warm water
½ tbsp crunchy peanut butter

We love Asian 'street food', especially Pad Thai. Unfortunately, living out in the English countryside, there's a distinct lack of Thai takeaways, which is why we had to learn to make our own healthy version. Well (after happily trialling hundreds of bowls) we're proud to say we cracked it with this fresh and clean dish that's easy to make and naturally high in protein and healthy fats.

1. Place the dried rice noodles in a large bowl and cover with boiling water. Leave to soften for 3 minutes then rinse with cold water and drain. Set aside.

2. Coat the base of a frying pan with spray light oil and lightly fry the shallots until soft then stir in the remaining sauce ingredients. Let the sauce bubble and only slightly reduce then pour into a bowl and set aside.

3. In the same pan, fry off the chicken strips until cooked through before adding the soaked rice noodles along with the spring onions and beansprouts.

4. Let the beansprouts soften slightly and the noodles heat up. Push everything to one side of the pan and add the beaten eggs to the empty side of the pan to gently scramble before mixing everything together.

5. Finally, add the pad thai sauce to the pan and mix everything together. Divide between two warmed plates, scatter over the roasted peanuts and squeeze over a wedge of lime to serve.

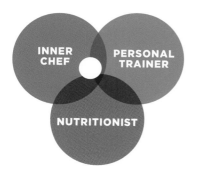

INNER CHEF
PERSONAL TRAINER
NUTRITIONIST

PLANT-BASED TACO CRUNCH WRAP

SERVES 5

Preparation time: 10 minutes
Cooking time: 30 minutes

FOR THE FILLING
2 peppers, finely diced
1 red onion, finely chopped
400g meat-free mince
1 tsp dried oregano
1 tsp cumin
1 tsp smoked paprika
1 tsp dried chilli powder
1 tsp dried chilli flakes
1 tsp celery salt
1 tsp onion powder
½ tsp garlic purée
1 tbsp agave syrup
2 tbsp no-added-sugar tomato
   ketchup
1 tbsp tomato purée
spray light oil for cooking

FOR THE SOUR CREAM
2 tsp soya milk
70g Violife cream cheese (or other
   plant-based soft cheese)

5 large wholemeal tortilla wraps
150g plant-based Cheddar-style
   cheese, grated
80g gem lettuce, finely
   shredded
10 cherry tomatoes, sliced
30g/1 bunch fresh coriander,
   chopped
1 lime, cut into wedges

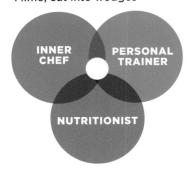

INNER CHEF

PERSONAL TRAINER

NUTRITIONIST

Presenting the very best of plant-powered recipes. This fully loaded taco wrap has a sweet chilli, meat-free mince filling that's high in protein, sprinkled with plant-based Cheddar-style cheese, topped with fresh leafy greens and juicy tomato, drizzled with your very own homemade sour cream, and all wrapped up in a wholemeal tortilla.

1. Preheat the oven to 200°C/180°C fan/gas 6 and line a baking tray with parchment paper.

2. Lightly coat the base of a large frying pan with spray light oil and cook the peppers, onion and mince over a medium-high heat for 5 minutes until the mince is brown and the peppers and onions have started to soften.

3. Stir in all the herbs and spices then add 300ml of water and leave the mince to simmer for a few minutes. Stir in the agave syrup, tomato ketchup and tomato purée and continue to simmer for a further 15 minutes to thicken up a little and for the flavours to develop.

4. Make the plant-based sour cream by mixing together the soya milk and cream cheese in a small bowl and set aside.

5. To assemble the taco parcels, divide the mince between the five wraps, placing it in the centre of each wrap. Top with the grated cheese, lettuce, tomatoes and coriander and finish with a drizzle of sour cream. Leave a generous border around the edge of each wrap to help make the folding easier.

6. Fold the edges of the tortilla in approximately 5 times until the filling is enclosed then quickly and carefully flip the wrap over so the folds are face down and no filling can escape.

7. Place the wraps on the lined baking tray and bake in the oven for 5 minutes until crispy and golden brown. Serve warm on a platter with the lime wedges.

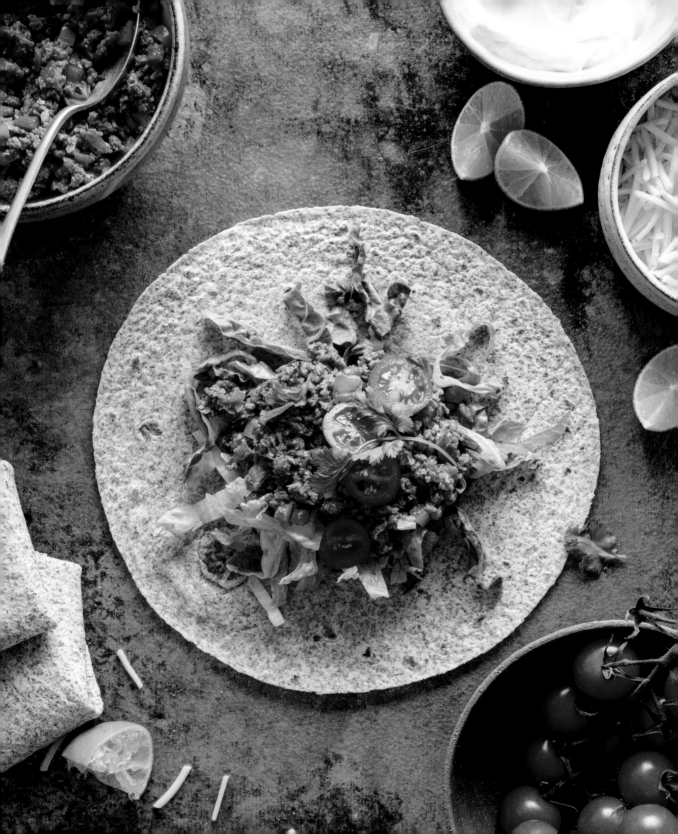

FALAFEL & BLACK RICE POKE BOWL

SERVES 2

Preparation time: 45 minutes + 24 hours soaking + 1 hour chilling
Cooking time: 50 minutes

125g dried chickpeas
30g/1 bunch fresh parsley, roughly chopped
30g/1 bunch fresh coriander, roughly chopped
½ tsp garlic purée
½ white onion, roughly chopped
1 tsp cumin
1 tbsp Thai green curry paste
plain flour, to thicken
½ tsp baking powder
sea salt and freshly ground black pepper
spray light oil for frying

FOR THE BUTTERNUT SQUASH MASH
½ butternut squash peeled, chopped and deseeded
100g carrots, peeled and chopped

There is a bit of preparation involved with this dish. However, if you are meal prepping for the week this is perfect, because there are so many different colours, textures and flavours going on – so you won't get bored! This plant-based poke bowl is one you'll look forward to again and again and is a great way to introduce a variety of vegetables into your diet. See the photo on the next page.

1. Place the dried chickpeas in a bowl of water, making sure the water comes to 5cm above the chickpeas, and soak for at least 24 hours.

2. Drain the chickpeas well then add to a food processor with the parsley, coriander, garlic purée and onion. Blitz to a coarse crumb then transfer to a bowl and stir through the cumin, Thai green curry paste and a good pinch each of salt and pepper. Cover the bowl and place in the fridge for an hour to firm up a little.

3. You want the falafel mixture to be crumbly but sticky so don't over process it. You may find you need to add a few teaspoons of plain flour if your mixture is too wet or a few teaspoons of water if it is too dry. Either way, add these a little at a time. You need the mixture to be a paste that you can squeeze together to form patties.

4. Place the butternut squash and carrots in a saucepan of boiling water and cook for 15 minutes until soft enough to mash. Drain, season to taste, then mash the carrots and squash until smooth and set aside.

5. Cook the black rice in a large pan of boiling water for 25–30 minutes until just tender. Drain and leave to cool slightly.

6. While the rice is cooking, remove the falafel mixture from the fridge and stir through the baking powder. Use your hands to roll the mixture into 10 golf-ball-sized balls then flatten them slightly to make little patties.

7. Heat a non-stick frying pan over a medium heat and cover the base with spray light oil. Place the falafel patties in the pan and cook on each side for about 3–4 minutes, until golden and crispy. (The edges of the patties won't really turn

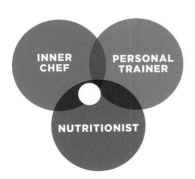

FOR THE LIME TAHINI YOGURT
100g plain soya yogurt
20g tahini paste
1½ tbsp lime juice

FOR THE SALAD
120g dried black rice
2 tsp sesame oil
30g spinach
30g kale
100g edamame beans
100g cooked beetroot, grated

the golden crispy colour as they are not fully submerged in oil, however, this is a healthier and more controlled cooking method if monitoring macros.)

8. When the falafel have cooked, remove from the pan and set aside. Wipe the pan with a piece of kitchen towel, add the 2 teaspoons of sesame oil and lightly fry the spinach and kale with a little salt and pepper to soften and darken the greens a little. This should only take a few minutes.

9. Mix the tahini yogurt ingredients together in a small bow and combine all the salad ingredients. Serve the yogurt alongside the falafel, mash, edamame beans, beetroot and salad.

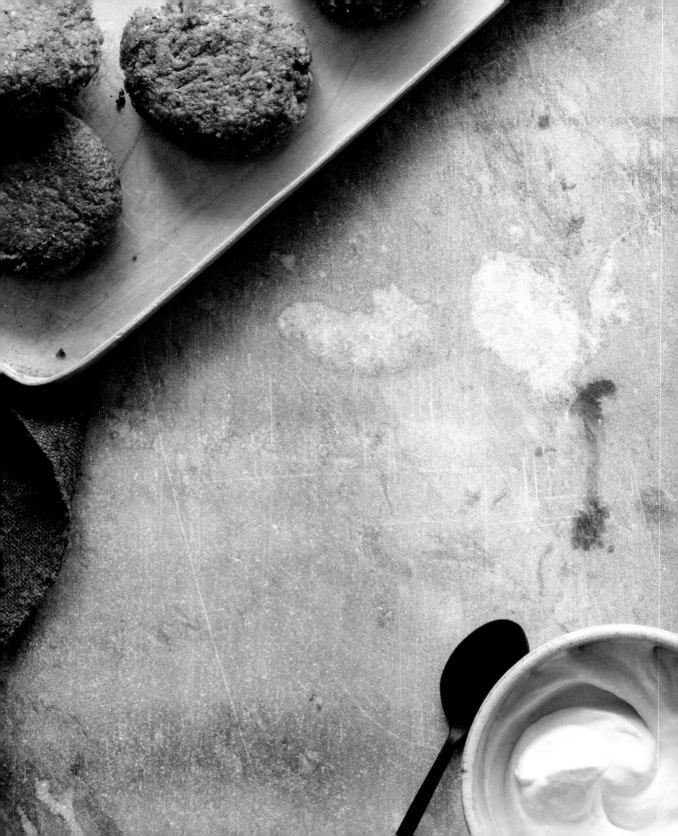

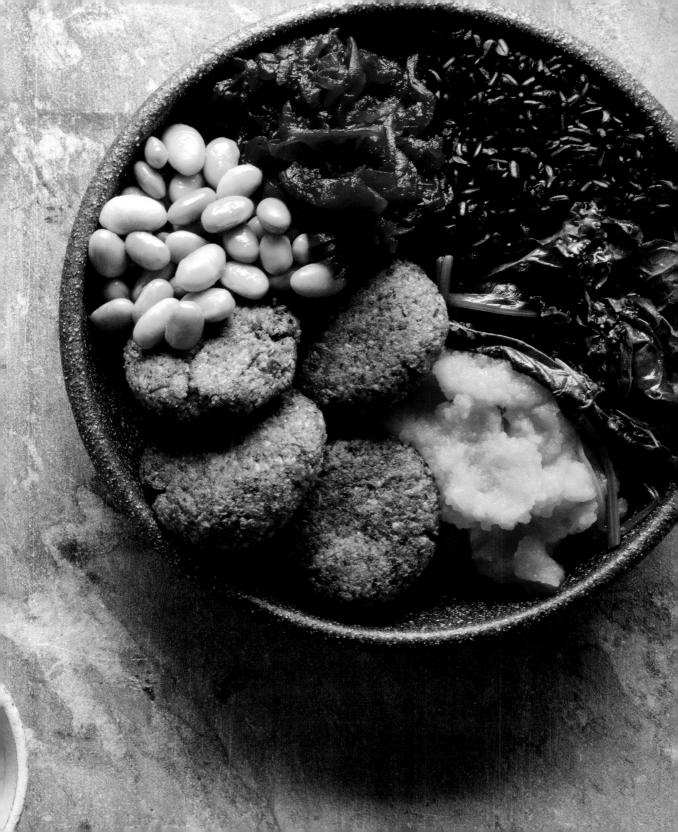

CALORIES 686
PROTEIN 55g
FAT 17g
CARBS 67g
SUGARS 11g

SERVES
2

LEMON CHICKEN & WHITE WINE SPAGHETTI

Preparation time: 10 minutes
Cooking time: 15 minutes

140g dried spaghetti, choose wholewheat pasta for a healthier option
1 shallot, thinly sliced
2 skinless chicken breasts, roughly chopped
80g baby plum tomatoes, halved
1 tsp garlic purée
100ml white wine
150ml Elmlea single light cream 45% less fat
juice of 1 lemon
7g/¼ bunch chives, finely chopped
15g/½ bunch parsley, roughly chopped
large handful of spinach
20g Parmesan, finely grated
sea salt and freshly ground black pepper
spray light oil for cooking

This is one of the quickest dinnertime recipes you will find in this book. Tender cooked pieces of chicken and soft, sweet, juicy plum tomatoes coated in a zingy lemon and white wine cream sauce, this recipe should be in everyone's proverbial bag of culinary tricks.

1. Cook the spaghetti in a large pan of salted boiling water for about 9 minutes until al dente.

2. While the pasta is cooking, lightly coat the base of a frying pan with spray light oil and fry the shallot over a medium heat until softened.

3. Add the chicken breast pieces to the shallot along with a pinch each of salt and pepper. As the chicken starts to brown add the tomatoes and the garlic purée. Once the chicken has fully cooked, add the white wine and let simmer for a few minutes to reduce slightly.

4. Add the cream, lemon juice, chives and parsley, let the sauce come to a simmer then turn off the heat immediately. Add a large handful of spinach and stir into the sauce to help it wilt.

5. Drain the spaghetti and fold it into the sauce then divide between two warmed pasta bowls. Grate a little Parmesan over to serve.

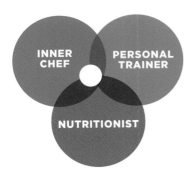

INNER CHEF — PERSONAL TRAINER — NUTRITIONIST

CALORIES 602
PROTEIN 59g
FAT 21g
CARBS 45g
SUGARS 20g

SERVES
4

TURKEY & CASHEW PASANDA

Preparation time: 10 minutes
Cooking time: 25 minutes

500g skinless turkey breast
   steaks, diced
4 flatbreads

FOR THE PASANDA SAUCE
1 white onion, finely diced
6 cardamom pods, crushed and
   seeds removed
1½ tsp ground cinnamon
1 tsp garam masala
¼ tsp ground cumin
½ tsp sweet paprika
1 tsp garlic purée
1 tsp ginger purée
1 tsp onion powder
½ tbsp tomato purée
50g cashew nuts
300ml chicken stock
100g fat-free yogurt
100ml reduced-fat sour cream
1 tbsp honey
20g flaked almonds, toasted
50g dried cranberries
a small bunch fresh coriander,
   leaves picked and finely
   chopped
spray light oil for cooking

We love a creamy curry, and among the many versions we've trialled, tested and tasted it's this homemade pasanda that comes out on top. Our version is cashew-based, giving the sauce covering the tender turkey pieces the most milky, sweet flavour. This, along with the crunch from the flaked almonds and sweetness from the cranberries, make this hands-down our favourite curry dish.

1. Coat the base of a large saucepan with spray light oil, set over a medium heat and sweat the onion for a few minutes before adding the cardamom seeds, cinnamon, garam masala, cumin, paprika, garlic, ginger, onion powder and tomato purée. Continue cooking until the onions are soft and the spices are fragrant. (If you're worried the onions are catching you can always add a small splash of water.)

2. Add the diced turkey and fry until fully cooked through.

3. Place the cashews in a food processor and pulse for a few seconds at a time until they are fine and evenly ground. Add the ground cashews and stir before adding the chicken stock. Let the sauce simmer for a few minutes to thicken slightly.

4. Finally, add the yogurt, sour cream and honey and stir everything together.

5. Briefly toast the flatbreads to warm them through. Divide the pasanda between four warmed plates then scatter over the flaked almonds, cranberries and coriander. Serve with the warm flatbreads.

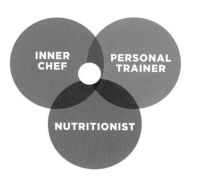

INNER CHEF

PERSONAL TRAINER

NUTRITIONIST

CALORIES 522
PROTEIN 42g
FAT 19g
CARBS 40g
SUGARS 11g

SERVES 4

SWEET PEPPER & HARISSA LAMB KEBABS WITH SHIRAZI SALAD

Preparation time: 20 minutes
Cooking time: 40 minutes

500g minced lamb
100g peppers (any colour), finely chopped
1 red onion, finely chopped
1 tsp smoked paprika
1 tsp garlic purée
1 tsp harissa smoky paste
½ tbsp dried parsley
2 eggs
sea salt and freshly ground black pepper

FOR THE SHIRAZI SALAD
5 tomatoes, diced
1 cucumber, diced
2 red onions, finely diced
6 tbsp lemon juice
1 tbsp dried mint
2 tbsp fresh coriander, roughly chopped

TO SERVE
4 wholemeal pita breads
0%-fat Greek yogurt (optional)

For this recipe, we took the very best of Middle Eastern cuisine and added a twist in the form of smoky harissa-flavoured lamb kebabs and a juicy, citrus herby salad. When stuffed into a pita bread it tastes incredible and, in many ways, is a cleaner and healthier version of the original that helps you meet your protein requirements for the day.

1. Place all the kebab ingredients in a large mixing bowl and season with salt and pepper. With clean hands, knead the ingredients to mix them together. Cover the bowl and place in the fridge for at least 5 hours to marinate and let the flavours develop.

2. To make the salad, place all the salad ingredients in a large mixing bowl and mix together with a spoon. Season to taste and place in the fridge until you are ready to serve.

3. Preheat the oven to 200°C/180°C fan/gas 6.

4. Press the lamb mixture into a loaf tin and spread it out evenly. Place in the preheated oven for 35–40 minutes or until cooked through. Turn the lamb out onto a board and cut into quarters then slice each quarter into three pieces.

5. Just before you serve, pop the pita breads in a toaster so they are nice and warm. To serve, stuff the shirazi salad and lamb kebab into the toasted pita breads, adding a dollop of Greek yogurt if you like.

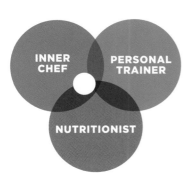

INNER CHEF

PERSONAL TRAINER

NUTRITIONIST

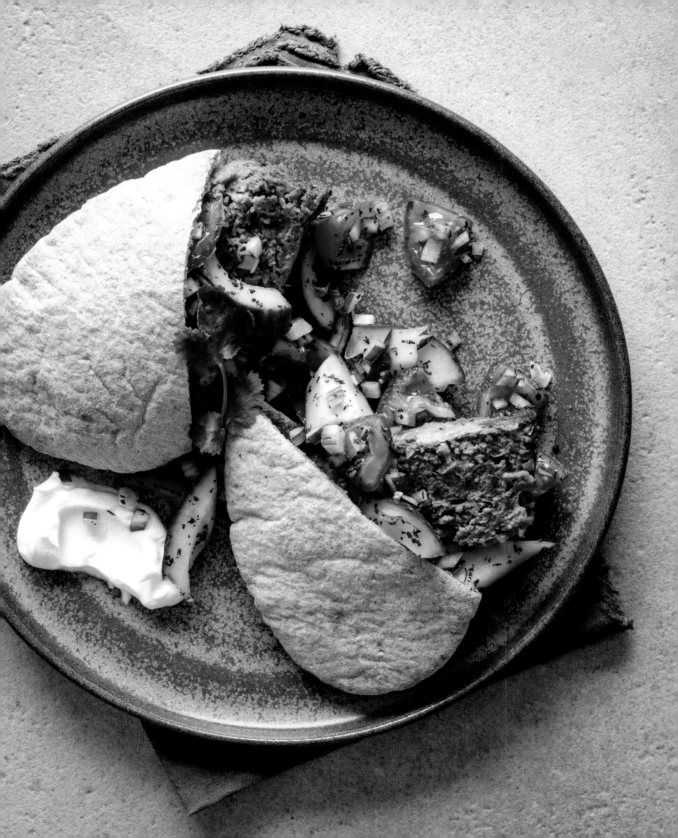

CALORIES 1047
PROTEIN 96g
FAT 42g
CARBS 72g
SUGARS 34g

SERVES
2

DOUGHNUT BURGER

Preparation time: 20 minutes
Cooking time: 20 minutes

FOR THE BURGER PATTY
1 white onion, finely diced
1 red onion, finely diced
500g lean minced beef
½ tsp onion powder
½ tsp garlic powder
2 tsp smoked paprika
sea salt and freshly ground
    black pepper
spray light oil for cooking

TO SERVE
4 slices smoked back bacon
4 slices Red Leicester cheese
4 ringed doughnuts
25g pickled gherkins
2 tomato slices

If we forget about calories and throw nutritional science out the window (just for a second), then this is hands down my favourite recipe in this book. Whether you're having a dirty bulk, a 'cheat meal' or you just need a colossal number of calories for a mammoth endurance expedition, this is the greatest culinary creation you will ever try. Creating it is so simple, too! Find your favourite doughnuts and then 'sandwich' numerous layers of homemade caramelised onion beef patties, Red Leicester cheese, sliced gherkins and smoked back bacon in between them. Once done, sit back and devour it. If you're being more considerate of your nutritionals, simply halve the ingredients of the burger patty and serving suggestions for a less-calorific treat.

1. Heat a large frying pan over a medium heat and cover the base with spray light oil. Fry the onion for a few minutes until soft and slightly caramelised.

2. Place the fried onions in a mixing bowl and add the remaining beef patty ingredients, along with a good pinch each of salt and pepper, and knead together until all the ingredients are fully combined. Use your hands to mould two even patties, making sure they are just a little bigger than your doughnut as they will shrink when cooking.

3. Add a little extra spray oil to the pan used to cook the onions and cook the burgers for 4–5 minutes on each side until cooked through (reduce the cooking time a little if you like your burgers pink in the middle.) When you have flipped your burgers, add the bacon to the same pan and cook for a few minutes until crispy.

4. Just before the burgers are done, place a cheese slice on top of each burger and place a lid on the frying pan for a few minutes until the cheese has melted.

5. Now you can start to build your burger! Place the cheese-topped beef patties on the bottom doughnuts then top with the smoked bacon, gherkins and tomato before placing the the other doughnuts on top to finish what can only be described as a masterpiece!

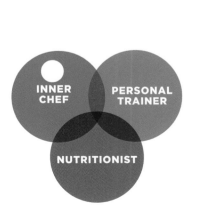

INNER CHEF

PERSONAL TRAINER

NUTRITIONIST

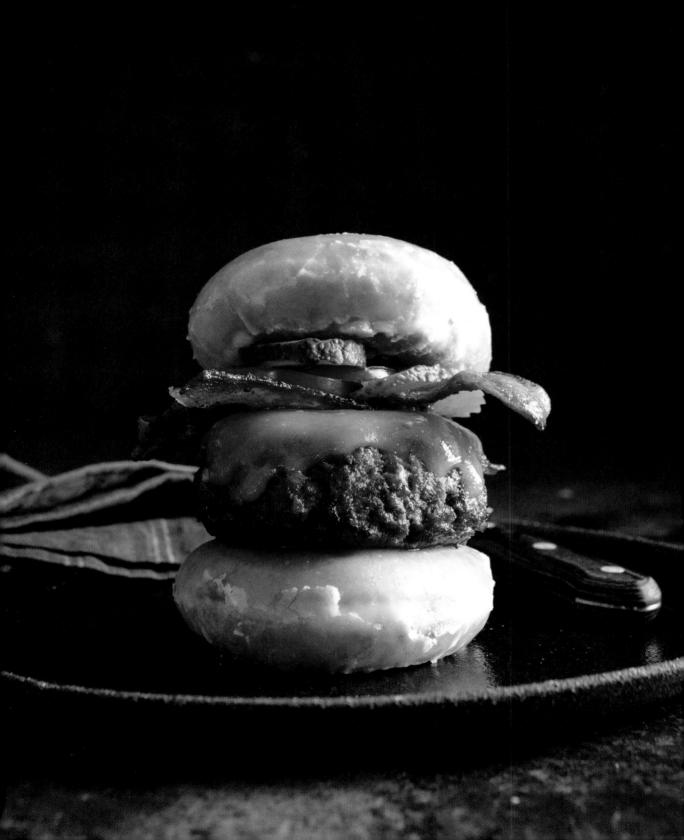

CALORIES 395
PROTEIN 42g
FAT 7g
CARBS 35g
SUGARS 7g

SERVES 6

CREAMY GREENY CHICKEN FILO PIE

Preparation time: 30 minutes
Cooking time: 20 minutes

2 white onions, diced
5 skinless chicken breasts, chopped into 3-cm chunks
½ tsp ground white pepper
300g leeks, sliced
200g frozen peas
200g frozen green beans
1 tsp garlic purée
2 tsp dried thyme
1 chicken stock cube
50g 50% reduced-fat crème fraiche
180g Philadelphia Lightest cream cheese (or other low-fat cream cheese)
200g pack of filo pastry
spray light oil for cooking

Chicken pie is a real comfort food, especially this one, with the tenderness of chicken pieces, and the sweetness and textures of the leeks, peas and green beans, all folded in with a creamy cheesy sauce. The reason this recipe is so good is because it can be prepared in advance and is perfect for eating with others, allowing you to enjoy a meal with friends that isn't going to make you fall out of your macros for the day.

1. Preheat the oven to 190°C/170°C fan/gas 5.

2. Lightly coat the base of a large saucepan with spray light oil and sauté the onions over a medium heat until soft and just starting to brown. Add the chicken to the pan along with the white pepper and a pinch of salt and cook for a few more minutes.

3. Add the leeks, peas, green beans, garlic purée and dried thyme and mix well, then let the vegetables soften for 5 minutes.

4. Mix the stock cube with 400ml of boiling water and stir well before adding to the pan. Bring the mixture to the boil and immediately reduce the heat to a simmer for 10 minutes.

5. On a very low heat, stir in the crème fraiche and cream cheese then pour the chicken pie filling into a deep baking dish. (I use a 33 x 23 x 7-cm ceramic dish, but anything will work as long as the filling fits!)

6. Gently scrunch up each sheet of filo pastry and place on top of the filling until the surface is fully covered. (There is no right or wrong way to do this, each time you make it, the appearance will be slightly different.) Spray the filo with a little spray light oil and bake the pie for 20 minutes or until the filo sheets are golden and crispy.

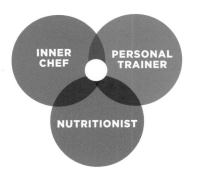

INNER CHEF

PERSONAL TRAINER

NUTRITIONIST

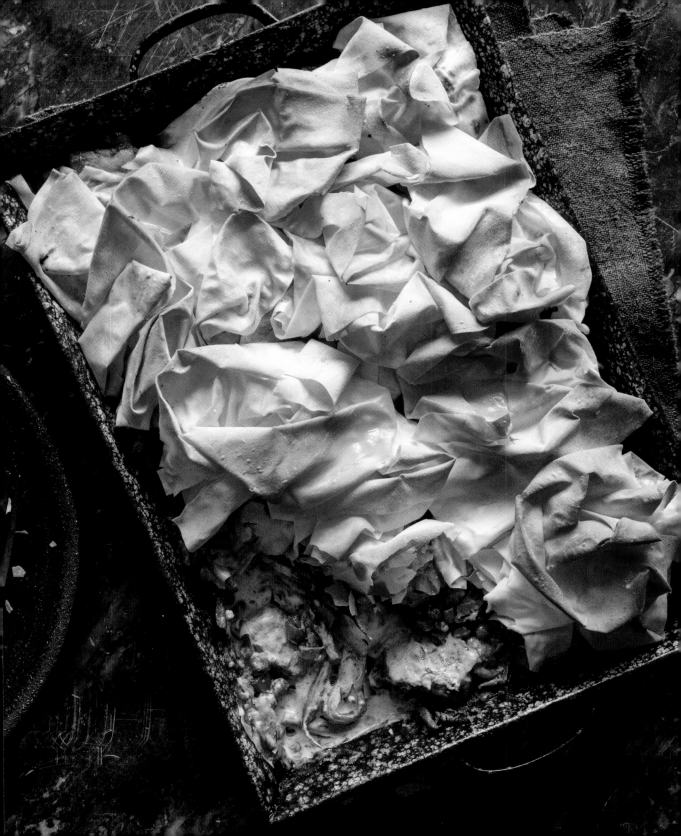

CALORIES 461
PROTEIN 41G
FAT 8G
CARBS 55G
SUGARS 14G

SERVES 2

MISO-GLAZED COD RAMEN

Preparation time: 15 minutes +
    2 hours marinating
Cooking time: 20 minutes

250g/2 cod fillets
½ tsp white miso paste
1 tbsp mirin
1 tbsp light soy sauce
1 tsp ginger purée
1 tsp sesame oil

FOR THE RAMEN
1 tsp chilli oil
½ tsp white miso paste
½ tsp garlic purée
1 tsp ginger purée
6 spring onions, sliced
2 vegetable stock cubes
½ tbsp light soy sauce
½ tbsp fish sauce
120g fine egg noodles
100g pak choi

TO GARNISH
3 spring onions, sliced
30g tinned bamboo shoots

This recipe almost defies the laws of gastronomy and dietetics with how much flavour it packs into each dish versus the calories you're actually consuming. A miso-glazed cod fillet, pak choi and bamboo shoots on top of a bed of noodles and all swimming in a light vegetable broth, scattered with spring onions and a little chilli oil. It's perfect as a light lunch when you've an afternoon or evening training session still to come.

1. Place the cod fillets in a mixing bowl with the white miso paste, mirin, soy sauce, ginger purée and sesame oil. Give everything a stir, making sure the cod is completely coated in the marinade and place in the fridge for an hour to marinate.

2. Heat the grill to medium-high and place the marinated fish on a foil-lined baking tray. Cook under the grill for 10 minutes until the marinade has crisped up a little and the cod is perfectly flaky.

3. Meanwhile, make the ramen by frying the chilli oil, miso paste, garlic purée, ginger purée and spring onions in a large saucepan over a medium heat for 2 minutes. Add the vegetable stock cubes along with 500ml of boiling water and stir in the soy and fish sauces. Bring the broth to the boil while stirring to help the stock cubes break down, then reduce the heat to a simmer. Simmer for a few minutes then add the noodles and cook for 3 minutes, stirring occasionally, then add the pak choi. Cover the pan with a lid and cook for a further 5 minutes or until the pak choi has wilted.

4. Serve the ramen in large bowls and top with the miso cod. Garnish with some sliced spring onions and the bamboo shoots.

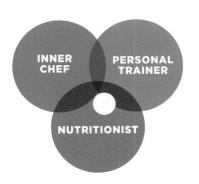

INNER CHEF
PERSONAL TRAINER
NUTRITIONIST

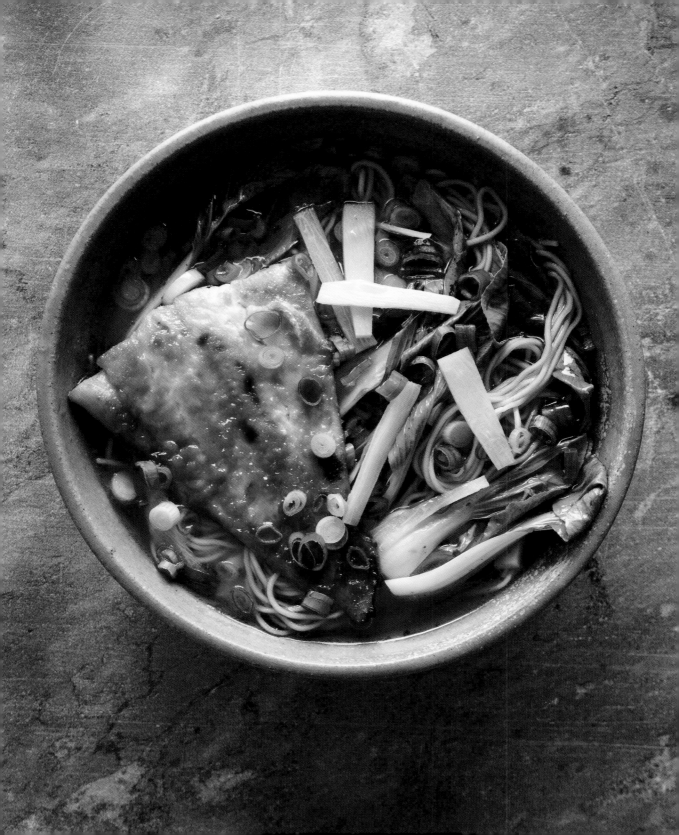

CALORIES 646
PROTEIN 27g
FAT 36g
CARBS 70g
SUGARS 20g

SERVES 4

TOFU RAISUKAREE

Preparation time: 20 minutes +
1 hour for pressing the tofu
Cooking time: 30 minutes

400g firm tofu
4 tbsp light soy sauce
½ tsp garlic powder
1 tbsp sesame oil

FOR THE SAUCE
2 red onions, finely chopped
2 tsp garlic purée
60g red Thai curry paste
2 tbsp fish sauce
juice of 2 limes
400g tin reduced-fat coconut
  milk
1 vegetable stock cube
400g mangetout
6 spring onions, chopped
2 peppers, sliced
1 green chilli, deseeded and
  finely chopped
20g/⅔ bunch fresh coriander,
  roughly chopped

TO SERVE
200g Tenderstem broccoli
500g microwaveable basmati
  rice

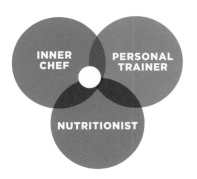

INNER CHEF
PERSONAL TRAINER
NUTRITIONIST

This Thai red curry has a pleasant hit of spice, combined with a citrusy fresh flavour. It's so versatile, the tofu can be swapped for pretty much anything – chicken, prawns, turkey, beef, you name it. Packed with 27g of protein per serving. Depending on your training goals, this recipe could be perfect for you.

1. Place the tofu on a clean tea towel and cut into chunks (I cut three ways on the short side and four ways on the long side.) Leaving the tofu in a block, carefully wrap the tea towel over the tofu and place a chopping board on top. Weight the board with a couple of weights – tins of beans are perfect for this job! This will help to remove excess water from the tofu. Leave the tofu to press for 30 minutes to 1 hour.

2. Preheat the oven to 200°C/180°C fan/gas 6 and line a baking tray with parchment paper.

3. Mix the soy sauce, garlic powder and sesame oil together in a bowl. Gently stir the tofu through the soy mix, and when coated place each piece of tofu onto the lined baking tray. Bake the tofu in the oven for 20 minutes, until nice and crunchy.

4. When the tofu is nearly baked, lightly fry the onion, garlic purée and curry paste in a large saucepan over a medium heat, until the onions are soft. Add the fish sauce, lime juice and coconut milk and gently stir in the vegetable stock cube until dissolved. When the curry begins to simmer, add the mangetout, spring onions, peppers and green chilli and let the vegetables soften slightly, being careful not to let the curry come above a simmer.

5. Cook the Tenderstem in a small pan of boiling water for 3–4 minutes and prepare the rice according to the packet instructions. Serve the curry, rice and broccoli in a bowl, top with the crispy tofu and finish by sprinkling over some chopped coriander.

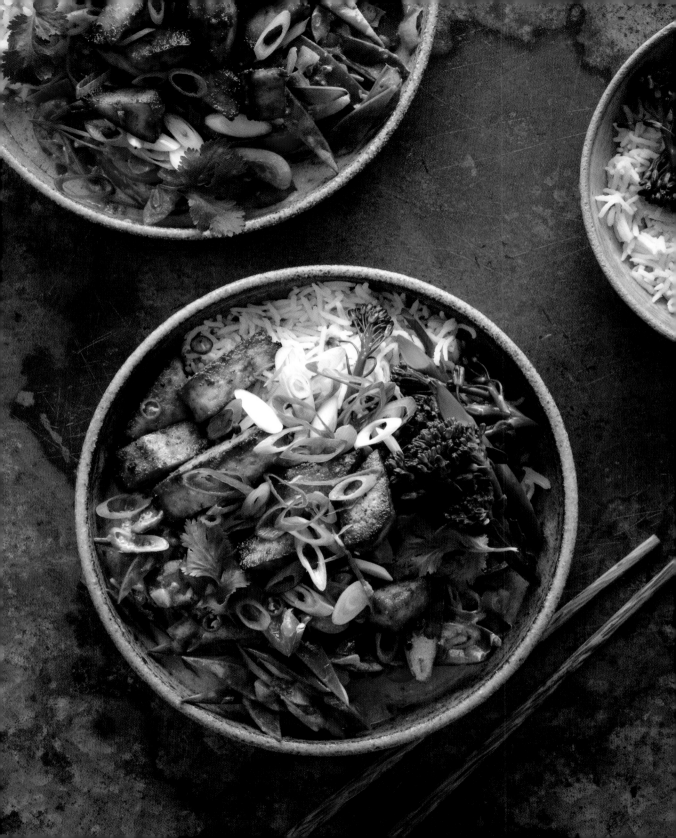

CALORIES 1115
PROTEIN 80g
FAT 69g
CARBS 42g
SUGARS 41g

SERVES 4

GLAZED HONEY & MUSTARD BEEF SHORT RIBS

Preparation time: 5 minutes
Cooking time: 7 hours
   15 minutes

1.3kg beef short ribs
150g clear honey
50g wholegrain mustard

This recipe is made pretty much every other weekend in our house (it's basically a tradition). Cooked to perfection after years of testing, trialling and tasting, the tender melt-in-your-mouth beef has a crispy sweet and naturally salty edge that can be used in many types of meals. In summer, we usually pair this with a fresh, crunchy salad, and in the winter we cosy up for a Sunday roast with all the trimmings. Obviously, this is not the best recipe if you're monitoring your calorie intake, but it's amazing if you're bulking up or just want to meet your elevated protein requirements for the day. We say it serves four as we like hearty portions in this house, but it can be divided into more servings.

1. Preheat the oven to 160°C/140°C fan/gas 2.

2. Place the beef short ribs in a large oven dish with the bone side facing upwards and pour boiling water over to cover most of the meat. Wrap the oven dish in aluminium foil and place in the preheated oven for 6 hours, then turn the temperature up to 200°C/180°C fan/gas 6 and cook for a further hour.

3. In a small bowl, mix the honey and mustard together. Carefully take the short rib dish out of the oven and remove the ribs from the water. Place the ribs into a smaller baking dish, bone side down. By this stage, the short ribs should have shrunk through cooking. Trim off any excess fat from the meat now, if you prefer, but this is optional.

4. Pour the honey and mustard glaze onto the short ribs and place them back in the oven for 15 minutes until the honey glaze starts to caramelise. When the meat has crisped up around the sides a little it's ready to serve.

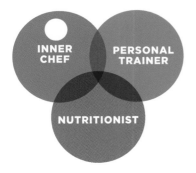

INNER CHEF

PERSONAL TRAINER

NUTRITIONIST

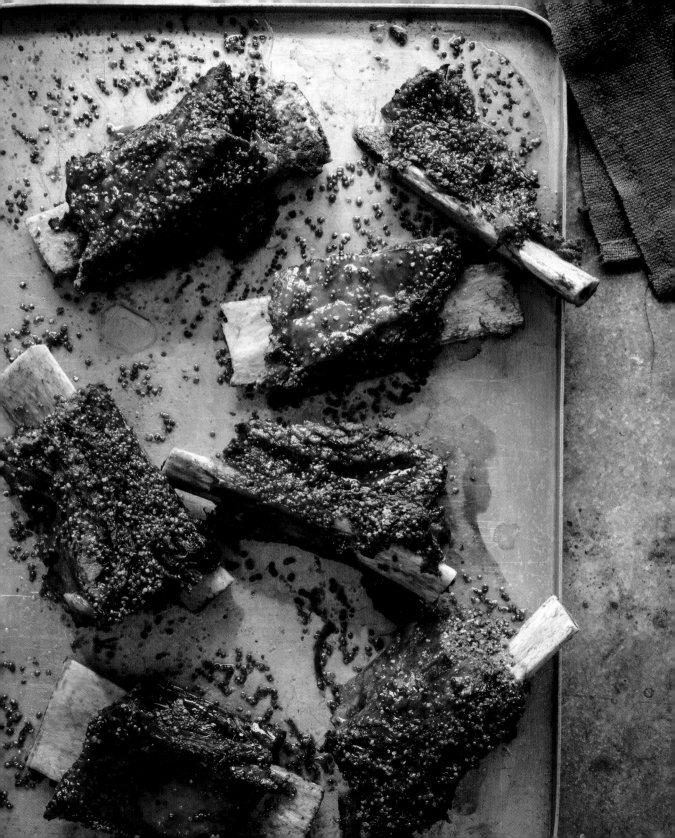

CALORIES 632
PROTEIN 83g
FAT 28g
CARBS 8g
SUGARS 6g

SERVES 2

Preparation time: 10 minutes
Cooking time: 25 minutes

3 chicken chipolata sausages
10g pine nuts
1½ tbsp harissa paste
50g feta cheese, crumbled
2 large chicken breasts
20g spinach
4 serrano ham slices

TO SERVE
100g baby plum tomatoes, halved
100g Tenderstem broccoli, sliced
½ red onion, sliced
1 tsp chilli oil
10g pine nuts

CHICKEN BREAST STUFFED WITH HARISSA FETA SAUSAGE STUFFING

This recipe is perfect if you're wanting something a little more special. A tender, succulent chicken breast, wrapped in serrano ham, with the rich flavours of smoky harissa sausage stuffing combined with the sharp feta cheese and crunchy pine nuts. Served with punchy chilli veg, this is one of the highest protein-packed recipes in the entire book.

1. Preheat the oven to 180°C/160°C fan/gas 4 and line a baking tray with parchment paper.

2. Squeeze the sausage meat from the skins into a small mixing bowl and use a fork to mix in the pine nuts, harissa paste and feta cheese.

3. Cut a slit along each chicken breast and stuff them with the harissa sausage mix and the spinach. Don't be afraid to pack it right in!

4. Using two ham slices for each chicken breast, wrap the ham around the chicken.

5. Place the chicken on the lined baking tray and cook for 25 minutes until the chicken is cooked through (the meat should have no hint of pinkness and the juices should run clear when gently pressed).

6. When the chicken has nearly finished cooking, gently fry the tomatoes, broccoli and red onion in the chilli oil for 5 minutes until the onions have softened and the broccoli is just tender.

7. Serve the chicken breasts with the vegetables and a final sprinkling of pine nuts.

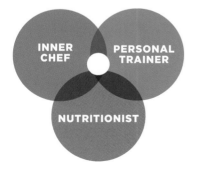

INNER CHEF
PERSONAL TRAINER
NUTRITIONIST

CALORIES 602
PROTEIN 24g
FAT 28g
CARBS 61g
SUGARS 30g

SERVES 2

Preparation time: 10 minutes
Cooking time: 25 minutes

4 pork and apple sausages
150g carrots, roughly chopped
200g swede, peeled and
   roughly chopped
200g sweet potato, peeled
   and roughly chopped
300g frozen garden peas
20g chicken gravy granules
sea salt and freshly ground
   black pepper

BANGERS & ROOT MASH

If you're wanting a faster, simpler, lower-calorie alternative to a roast dinner, then this is the ideal recipe for you. A whole plate of sweet root mash that's seasoned to perfection is then paired with fruity pork and apple sausages, sweet garden peas and covered with lashings of gravy to provide a high-carb, high-protein meal to fuel even the most intense workouts.

1. Preheat the oven to 200°C/180°C fan/gas 6 and line a baking tray with parchment paper.

2. Place the sausages on the lined baking tray and cook for 25 minutes until golden brown and piping hot throughout.

3. Meanwhile, place the carrots, swede and sweet potato in a large saucepan, cover with boiling water and simmer for 15 minutes until the vegetables are soft.

4. Meanwhile, simmer the peas in a separate saucepan for a few minutes then drain and set aside.

5. Drain the vegetables and roughly mash them before seasoning, to taste. (We like ours roughly mashed as we quite like the chunky texture, but just keep mashing if you prefer a smoother mash.)

6. Make the gravy by adding about 250ml of boiling water to the gravy granules and stirring until smooth. Add more boiling water if necessary to achieve the desired consistency.

7. Serve the bangers and mash in a bowl with the sweet root mash on the bottom, followed by two sausages, a splash of gravy and lots of peas on top.

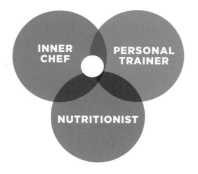

INNER CHEF
PERSONAL TRAINER
NUTRITIONIST

One-pot Wonders

Every one-pot wonder recipe in this book
is loaded with taste, texture and tradition.
Inspired by cultures from across the world,
the Persian-Brazilian stews, Tuscan pasta
and barbecue beef brisket recipes can only
be described as wholesome home cooking
at its very best.

CALORIES 718
PROTEIN 49g
FAT 38g
CARBS 42g
SUGARS 15g

SERVES 10

BBQ PULLED PORK BURGERS

Preparation time: 30 minutes
Cooking time: 7 hours
    30 minutes

1 red onion, diced
1 chicken stock cube, crumbled
200ml boiling water
200ml apple cider vinegar
200g BBQ sauce
1 tbsp smoked paprika
1 tbsp mild chilli powder
1 tbsp wholegrain mustard
2kg pork shoulder joint
sea salt and freshly ground black
    pepper

FOR THE SLAW
400g celeriac, coarsely grated
300g red cabbage, thinly sliced
350g carrots, coarsely grated
1 white onion, finely sliced
200g Lighter than Light
    mayonnaise
250g 0%-fat Greek yogurt
½ tsp celery salt powder
2 tbsp wholegrain mustard

TO SERVE
10 wholemeal buns
baby spinach leaves

The melt-in-your-mouth BBQ Pulled Pork Burger is one of the greatest burger-based creations to ever emerge from our kitchen and was inspired by the time I spent in America. Packed into a sweet bun and served with homemade slaw and greens, each mouthful is so smoky and juicy, since the pork has been slow-cooked in BBQ sauce and a combination of herbs and spices for hours.

1. Set a slow cooker on high.

2. Place all the pulled pork ingredients, apart from the pork joint, in the slow cooker along with a few good pinches each of salt and pepper and stir everything together. Add the pork joint and turn it over a few times to make sure it is fully coated. Leave to cook for 7 hours, turning the meat over halfway through the cooking time.

3. After 7 hours, the meat should be tender and readily fall apart. Take the joint out of the slow cooker and place on a chopping board to trim off any excess fat.

4. Use two forks to shred the meat then place the meat back in the slow cooker to cook for a further 30 minutes.

5. To make the slaw, mix the celeriac, red cabbage, carrots and onion together in a large bowl.

6. In a separate bowl, mix the mayonnaise, yogurt, celery salt and mustard together along with a big pinch each of salt and pepper. Add to the vegetables and mix together.

7. Serve the pork stuffed into the wholemeal buns, topped with the spinach leaves and a big spoonful of slaw on the side.

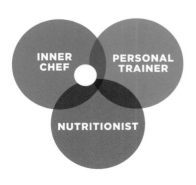

INNER CHEF

PERSONAL TRAINER

NUTRITIONIST

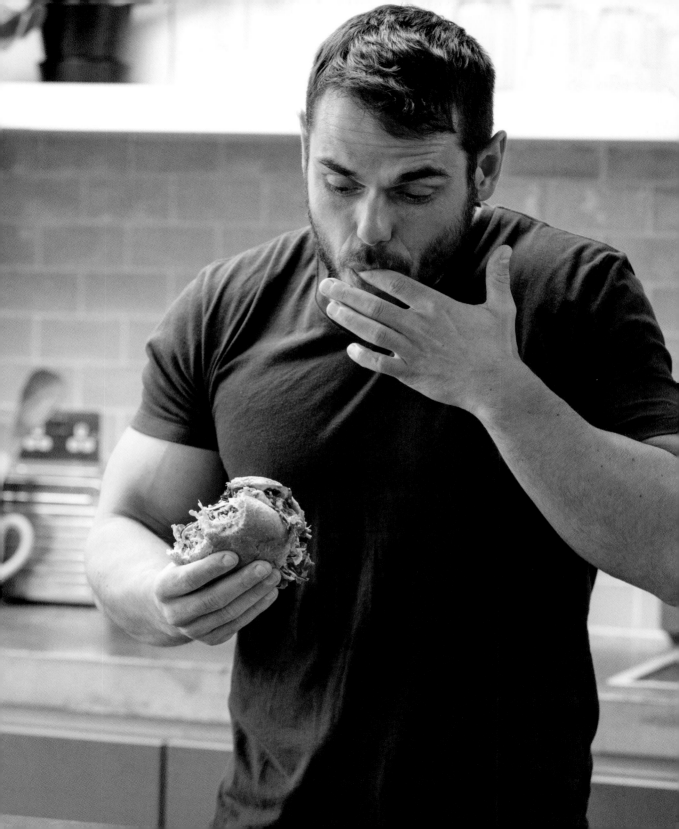

SERVES 4

BRAZILIAN BEAN STEW

Serves 4
Preparation time: 30 minutes +
  overnight soaking
Cooking time: 8 hours

FOR THE STEW
300g dried black turtle beans
200g dried yellow lentils
400g tin red kidney beans,
  drained and rinsed
1 red onion, diced
30g/1 bunch fresh coriander,
  roughly chopped
30g/1 bunch fresh parsley,
  roughly chopped
2 bay leaves
1 tsp chilli powder
1 tsp smoked paprika
½ tsp cayenne pepper
1 tsp ground coriander
1 tsp garlic purée
3 mixed coloured peppers,
  sliced
2 x 400g tins plum tomatoes
1 tsp chilli pepper purée
1 vegetable stock cube,
  dissolved in a splash of
  boiling water
1 tbsp balsamic vinegar
2 tbsp light soy sauce

There are many things I took from my time in Brazil, from a love of capoeira and samba music to a profound appreciation for the Amazon rainforest. But another thing I brought back was love for a Brazilian stew! Hester makes the most easy, wholesome, plant-based recipe as a mid-week tea that can also be used for meal preps throughout the week. It contains so many different textures and tastes, it can also easily be made into a meat dish by adding turkey meatballs.

FOR THE SALSA
4 vine tomatoes, chopped
1 red onion, finely chopped
2 tbsp lime juice
1 yellow pepper, diced into small
  chunks
15g/½ bunch fresh coriander,
  chopped
4 medium sweet potatoes
200g plant-based plain yogurt

1. Prepare the dried black beans by soaking them in a bowl of cold water overnight, making sure the water level is at least 2cm above the beans.

2. Place the soaked beans along with all the other stew ingredients in a slow cooker set on high and cook for 8 hours, stirring once halfway through the cooking time. And it's as simple as that! After 8 hours, all the beans and lentils should have cooked through and taken on the juices and flavours of the many herbs and spices they have been cooking in.

3. Prepare the salsa by mixing all the salsa ingredients together in a small salad bowl.

4. When you're ready to serve, heat the oven to 200°C/180°C fan/gas 6. Prick the sweet potatoes with a fork and place in a microwave to cook for 6 minutes. Place the cooked sweet potatoes in the oven, straight on the shelf, for 5–10 minutes to crisp up the skin.

5. Cut the sweet potatoes in half, spoon the flavoursome stew over the top and finish with a dollop of yogurt and a big spoonful of fresh salsa.

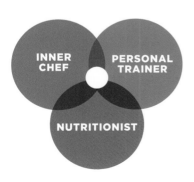

INNER CHEF
PERSONAL TRAINER
NUTRITIONIST

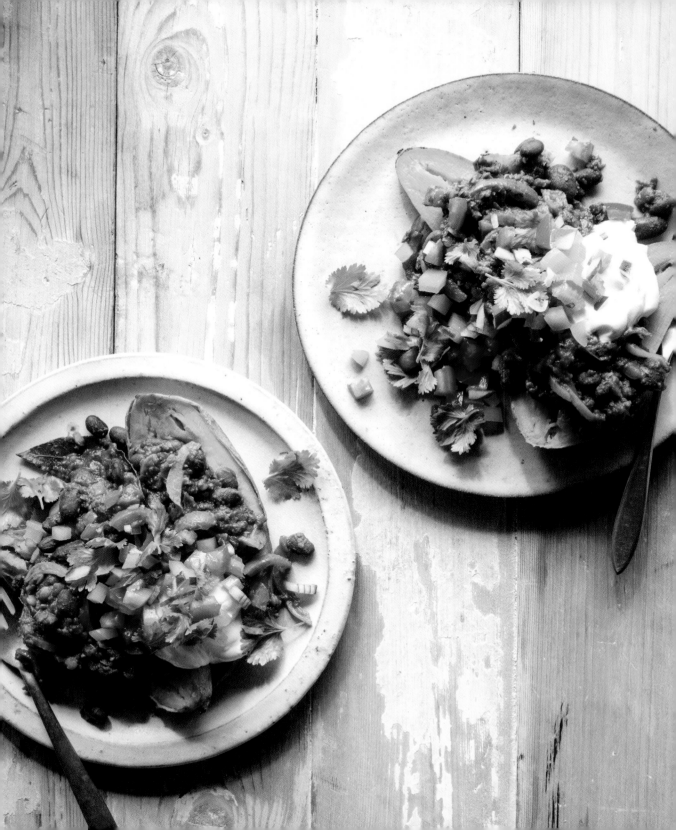

CALORIES 363
PROTEIN 49g
FAT 5g
CARBS 33g
SUGARS 11g

SERVES
4

PORK & TURKEY MEATBALL YELLOW LENTIL STEW (KHORESH GHEYMEH)

Preparation time: 20 minutes
Cooking time: 6 hours

2 x 400g tins chopped
   tomatoes
200g yellow lentils or split peas
¼ tsp ground cinnamon
1 tsp paprika
½ tsp turmeric
¼ tsp ground cumin
2 tbsp tomato purée
4 black dried limes
250g minced turkey
250g minced pork
2 white onions, finely chopped
sea salt and freshly ground
   black pepper
spray light oil for cooking

Khoresh Gheymeh, also known as Persian yellow lentil stew, is usually made with either beef or lamb. However, to reduce the fat content but still pack in the flavours, this recipe substitutes in white meats – lean turkey and pork. Traditionally, this dish is eaten with saffron rice, however, due to the lentils having a high carbohydrate content, sometimes we eat this with a side of fresh green stir-fried veg and a dollop of 0% fat yogurt.

1. Place the tinned tomatoes, 500ml of boiling water, the yellow lentils, cinnamon, paprika, turmeric, cumin, tomato purée and dried limes in a slow cooker.

2. Place the turkey and pork mince, one of the chopped onions and a pinch each of salt and pepper in a mixing bowl. Mix together with your hands and roll into 12 golf ball-sized balls.

3. Lightly coat a large frying pan with spray light oil and place over a medium heat. Fry the second chopped onion in the pan along with the 12 meatballs until lightly golden, turning the meatballs every so often to make sure they are evenly cooked. Once the meatballs have cooked on the outside, tip them into the slow cooker and stir in well to cover with the tomato sauce.

4. Set the slow cooker on high and cook for 6 hours. Then enjoy!

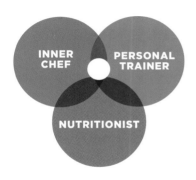

INNER CHEF PERSONAL TRAINER NUTRITIONIST

150 ONE-POT WONDERS

CALORIES 625
PROTEIN 65g
FAT 11g
CARBS 76g
SUGARS 7g

IRANIAN HERB STEW (GHORMEH SABZI)

SERVES 4

Preparation time: 40 minutes
Cooking time: 6 hours

1 white onion, finely chopped
750g beef, diced
1 tsp turmeric
1 beef stock cube
120g/4 bunches fresh parsley
90g/3 bunches fresh coriander
25g/1 bunch fresh chives
20g dried fenugreek leaves
4 black dried limes
400g tin red kidney beans, drained and rinsed
sea salt and freshly ground black pepper
spray light oil for cooking

FOR THE SAFFRON & BARBERRY RICE
300g white basmati rice
¼ tsp saffron threads
50g dried barberries or fresh pomegranate seeds
400ml chicken or vegetable stock

Hester and her family first introduced me to this Iranian national dish and I've been obsessed with it ever since. The beef is slowly cooked for hours with a selection of herbs and spices, juicy kidney beans and finally (the secret ingredient) dried limes. I can't describe another stew like this as the flavours are unique. A brilliant recipe for someone in search of high-protein alternatives. See photo on the next page.

1. In a frying pan over a medium heat, sauté the onion in some spray light oil until soft and translucent. Add the beef and turmeric with a pinch each of salt and pepper, and cook until the meat is sealed. Place in a slow cooker with the beef stock cube and 500ml of boiling water and set on high for 6 hours.

2. Wash the fresh herbs, pat dry and chop extremely finely – this is the most time-consuming bit, but it's worth it!

3. Coat a frying pan with spray light oil and sauté the chopped herbs and the dried fenugreek leaves over a low heat until dark in colour. This should take about 10–15 minutes. Add to the slow cooker and stir into the beef mixture.

4. After 5 hours, pierce the dried limes with a skewer or sharp knife to make tiny holes for the flavour to escape and place into the stew along with the kidney beans to cook for the remaining hour of cooking time.

5. To make the rice, rinse it in cold water in a sieve until the water runs clear – this may take a good few minutes.

6. Place the saffron in a small bowl and add 200ml of boiling water. Infuse for 10 minutes, to release its flavour and colour.

7. Coat a saucepan with spray light oil and fry the barberries over a medium heat to allow them to expand slightly. Add the rice to the barberry pan, stir to mix and coat the rice with the oil. Pour the saffron infusion over the rice then add the stock and a pinch of salt. Stir and bring to the boil.

8. Turn the heat down and simmer for 20 minutes, stirring to make sure the rice isn't sticking to the bottom of the pan.

9. When you're ready to serve the stew, fluff the rice with a fork and add a few extra barberries on top for decoration.

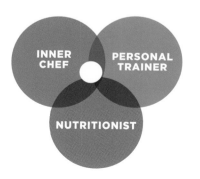

INNER CHEF
PERSONAL TRAINER
NUTRITIONIST

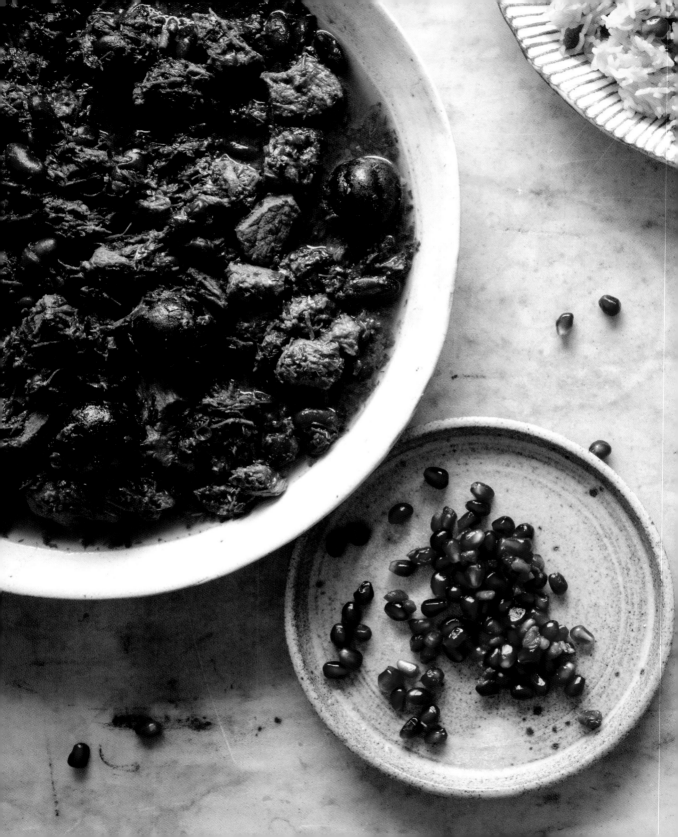

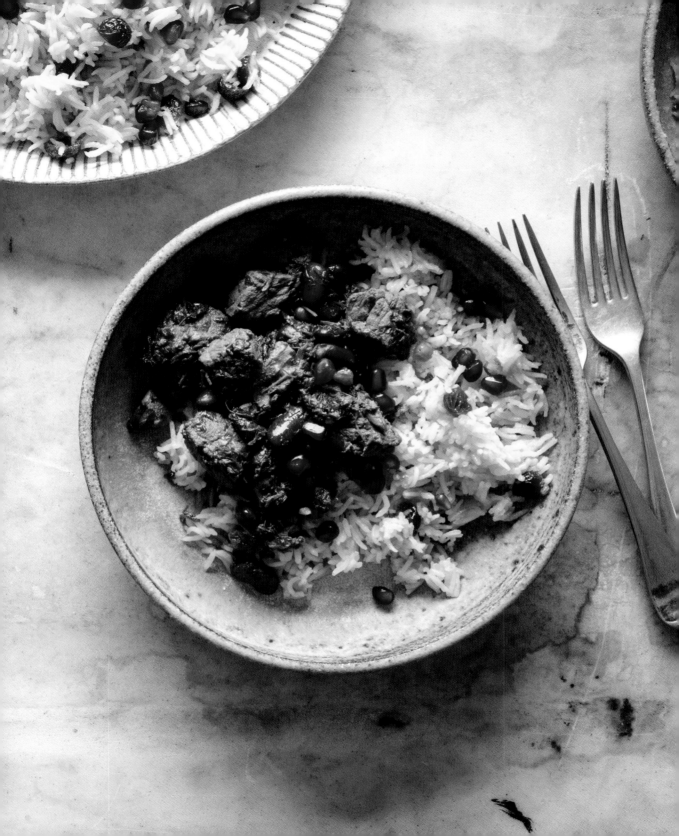

CALORIES 746
PROTEIN 48g
FAT 51g
CARBS 22g
SUGARS 11g

SERVES 6

CHICKEN, POMEGRANATE & WALNUT STEW (FESENJAN)

Preparation time: 20 minutes
Cooking time: 2 hours
    30 minutes

1 white onion, finely chopped
6 skinless chicken breasts
1 tbsp plain flour
300g walnuts, finely ground in
    a food processor
100g walnuts, chopped into
    small pieces
125ml pomegranate molasses
3 tbsp zero-calorie granulated
    white sugar replacer
1 chicken stock cube
¼ tsp ground cinnamon
¼ tsp freshly grated nutmeg
80g pomegranate seeds, to
    serve (optional)
sea salt and freshly ground
    black pepper
spray light oil for cooking

Persian food is packed with rich flavours, textures and tradition and is so often seasoned with an incredible array of spices and accompanied by pita bread or mountains of rice. This is why Hester (and all her family) are incredible cooks. But among all the dishes they've introduced me to, Persian Pomegranate Chicken (known as Fesenjan) stands out the most. Slowly cooked with toasted walnuts and pomegranate molasses; this earthy, rich, tangy and luscious stew bursts with Middle Eastern flavour and is best paired with a fresh juicy salad (Shirazi Salad see page 130) and a refreshing cucumber and mint yogurt (see page 156).

1. Lightly coat a frying pan with spray light oil and gently fry the onion over a medium heat until softened.

2. Roughly chop the chicken breasts and add to the onions along with a pinch each of salt and pepper. Make sure you seal the chicken on all sides, then turn the heat off and set aside.

3. In a separate pan, add the flour and both the ground and finely chopped walnuts over a medium heat. Cook for a few minutes until the mixture turns slightly darker in colour then add 1 litre of cold water. Stir constantly and slowly bring to the boil, this will take about 15-20 minutes. Lower the heat and let simmer for a couple of minutes.

4. Place both the walnut mixture and chicken mixture in a large, deep saucepan, along with the pomegranate molasses, sweetener, chicken stock cube, cinnamon and nutmeg. Set the pan over a medium heat and bring to the boil. Immediately turn down the heat to the lowest setting and let simmer for 2 hours, giving it a good stir every 30 minutes.

5. After 2 hours the stew will have become a rich, thick, dark consistency and when stirred the chicken will have broken down slightly with the tenderness. If the stew needs a little longer to thicken, leave on the heat for a little more time.

6. Serve with the pomegranate seeds and a fresh salad (see page 130 for a perfect Shirazi Salad Combo) along with a toasted pita bread or some rice.

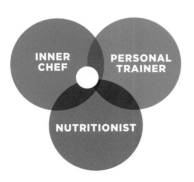

INNER CHEF

PERSONAL TRAINER

NUTRITIONIST

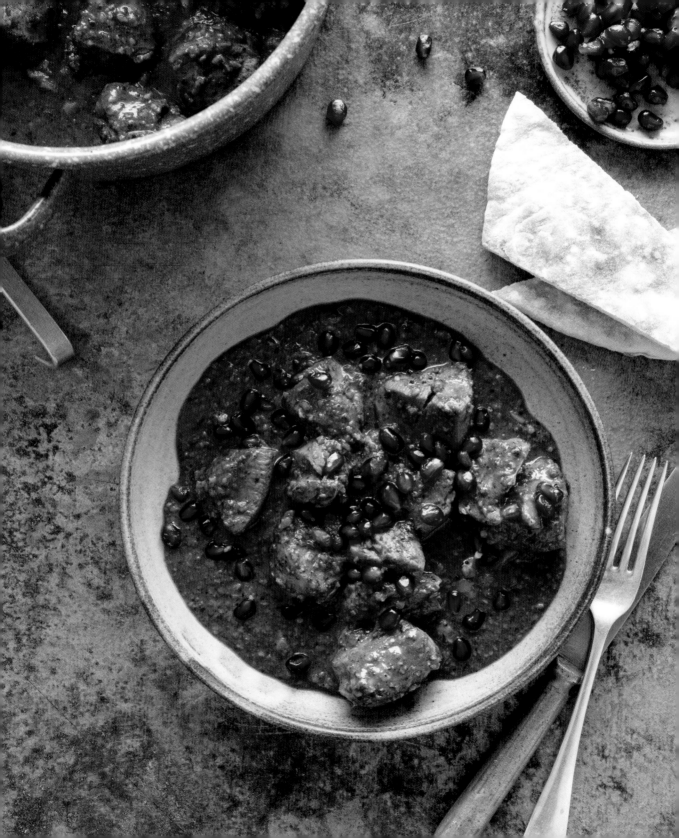

CALORIES 664
PROTEIN 56g
FAT 22g
CARBS 44g
SUGARS 6g

SERVES 4

CELERY & LAMB STEW (KHORESH KARAFS)

Preparation time: 20 minutes
Cooking time: 8 hours

100g/3 bunches fresh parsley
25g/1 bunch fresh mint
1 white onion, finely chopped
600g celery stalks, cut into
    4-cm pieces
700g diced lamb
½ tsp turmeric
4 black dried limes
4 wholemeal pita breads
sea salt and freshly ground
    black pepper
spray light oil for cooking

FOR THE YOGURT, CUCUMBER &
    MINT SAUCE
½ cucumber, coarsely grated
250g 0%-fat Greek yogurt
1 tsp dried mint
1 tsp dried dill

Persian celery stew (known as Khoresh Karafs) packs so much flavour into a single recipe, despite requiring relatively few ingredients. This high-protein dish is slow-cooked to perfection, so the tender pieces of lamb melt in your mouth and the juicy celery pieces take on all the flavours from the lime and mint. So easy to prepare, it's another great alternative if you're looking for a healthy stew with a difference.

1. Wash the fresh herbs, pat dry and chop very finely.

2. Place the chopped herbs in a frying pan with a little spray light oil over a low heat and sauté for 10–15 minutes until they have darkened in colour.

3. In a separate pan, sauté the onion and celery in some spray light oil until they begin to soften up. Add the diced lamb with the turmeric and a pinch each of salt and pepper and cook until the meat is fully sealed.

4. Place both the sautéed herb mix and the lamb mix in a slow cooker, add 500ml of boiling water and set on high for 8 hours.

5. After 6 hours, pierce the dried limes with a skewer or sharp knife to make tiny holes for the flavour to escape and place into the stew for the last 2 hours of cooking time.

6. To make the yogurt, cucumber and mint sauce, mix all the ingredients together and place in the fridge for 8 hours while the stew is cooking to ensure all the flavours infuse into the yogurt base.

7. Serve the stew and sauce with a toasted pita bread.

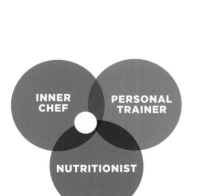

INNER CHEF

PERSONAL TRAINER

NUTRITIONIST

CALORIES 424
PROTEIN 50g
FAT 9g
CARBS 23g
SUGARS 15g

SIMPLE BEEF & RED WINE STEW

SERVES 4

Preparation time: 20 minutes
Cooking time: 6 hours

1 red onion, finely diced
500g beef, diced
1 tsp smoked paprika
1 courgette, halved lengthways
    and chopped
1 beef stock cube
½ tsp garlic purée
1 tsp dried thyme
500g carrots, roughly chopped
200g frozen peas
200g fine green beans
200ml red wine
20g gravy granules, to thicken
sea salt and freshly ground black
    pepper
spray light oil for cooking

A winter favourite, with chunky chopped vegetables that have taken on the rich, tender, meaty and red wine flavour. Either serve in a bowl for a low-carb meal option with a few greens or add your favourite side dish of creamy mash or roasted sweet potato wedges, like we do.

1. Coat a frying pan with spray light oil and lightly sauté the onion until soft and slightly brown. Add the diced beef, smoked paprika and a pinch each of salt and pepper and cook until the meat is fully sealed.

2. Add the courgette and let it soften slightly in the meat juices for a couple of minutes.

3. Place the meat mixture in a slow cooker along with the beef stock cube, 500ml of boiling water, garlic purée, thyme, carrots, peas and green beans and set on high for 6 hours.

4. Reusing the frying pan just used to seal the meat, pour in the red wine, bring to the boil and immediately turn down the heat to a simmer for a few minutes until it has reduced ever so slightly. Pour into the slow cooker and stir everything together.

5. Add the gravy granules to the stew 30 minutes before the end of the cooking time, stirring well so the stew thickens slightly.

6. Serve with some creamy mash or roasted sweet potato wedges.

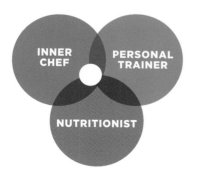

INNER CHEF

PERSONAL TRAINER

NUTRITIONIST

CALORIES 473
PROTEIN 36g
FAT 8g
CARBS 56g
SUGARS 18g

SERVES 3

TUSCAN SAUSAGE PASTA

Preparation time: 15 minutes
Cooking time: 5 hours

1 red onion, roughly chopped
100g celery, roughly chopped
200g carrots
8 low-fat chicken chipolata
 sausages, cut into medium-
 sized pieces
1 tsp dried basil
400g tin mixed beans, drained
 and rinsed
2 x 400g tins chopped
 tomatoes
1 tsp dried oregano
1 tsp rosemary
1 tsp garlic purée
1 tsp chilli pepper purée
1 tsp dried chilli flakes
2 tbsp balsamic vinegar
140g dried tagliatelle
20g Parmesan cheese, finely
 grated
sea salt and freshly ground
 black pepper
spray light oil for cooking

When your time is limited, cooking recipes that contain healthy whole foods can be difficult. But never fear, this Tuscan Sausage Pasta will come to your rescue. Easily prepped and refrigerated to be eaten when you need it, the calories and fat content of this traditional Italian dish have also been reduced by using chicken chipolata sausages rather than the beef that's conventionally used.

1. Coat a frying pan with the spray light oil and place over a medium heat. Sauté the onion, celery and carrots for 5 minutes until they start to caramelise. Add the chopped sausages and cook for a few minutes until the outsides are nice and golden.

2. Place the frying pan mixture, along with the rest of the ingredients, apart from the tagliatelle and Parmesan, in a slow cooker and set on high for 5 hours.

3. Fifteen minutes before the end of the cooking time, place the pasta in a pan of boiling salted water and cook for 10 minutes until al dente.

4. Drain the tagliatelle and add to the sausage stew, stirring well to allow the pasta to absorb the slow-cooked juices.

5. Season to taste and serve with a sprinkle of freshly grated Parmesan over the top.

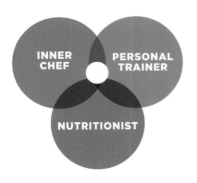

INNER CHEF
PERSONAL TRAINER
NUTRITIONIST

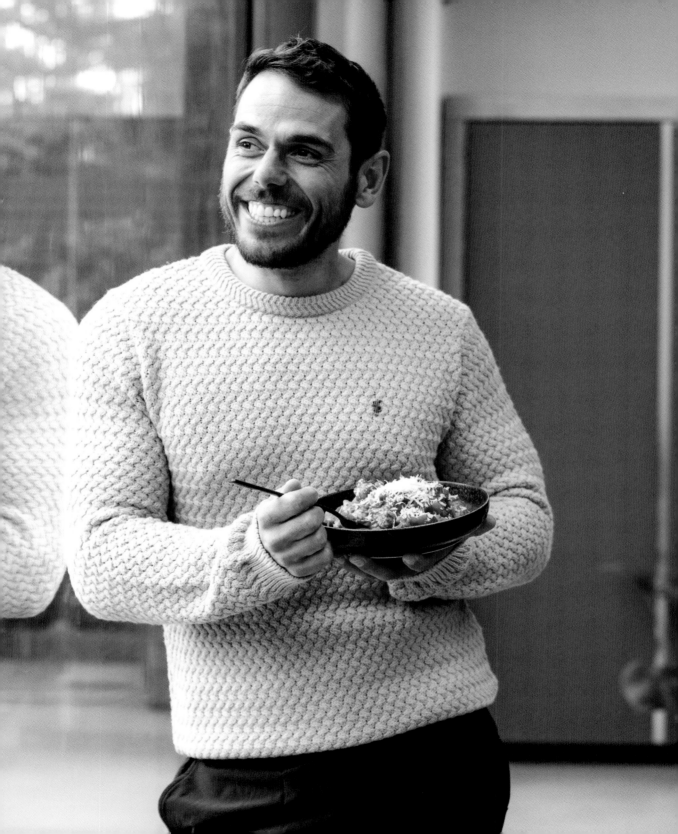

CALORIES 671
PROTEIN 52g
FAT 14g
CARBS 82g
SUGARS 26g

SERVES 4

ZESTY ORANGE & GINGER BEEF BRISKET ONE-POT

Preparation time: 20 minutes
Cooking time: 8 hours

1 white onion, finely chopped
500g beef brisket
500g carrots, roughly chopped
100g baby button mushrooms, halved
300ml pure orange juice
100ml red wine
1 tsp garlic purée
1 tsp ginger purée
1 beef stock cube
2 whole oranges
1 tsp cornflour
sea salt and freshly ground black pepper
spray light oil for cooking

FOR THE GARLIC BUTTERY POTATOES
800g white potatoes, peeled and chopped into large pieces
80g Flora Light spread (or other light spread)
1 tsp garlic purée
13g/½ bunch fresh parsley, finely chopped

One of the greatest recipes you can make in the autumn, this smells as good as it tastes. It's healthy, home comfort food at its best. Cooked slowly, the beef brisket falls off your fork and is full of rich, sweet, zesty flavour. It pairs perfectly with a hearty portion of garlic potatoes that are crispy on the outside, fluffy on the inside and glazed in butter. For a lower-carb alternative, this one-pot wonder serves brilliantly with just a few spring greens and Tenderstem broccoli.

1. Lightly coat a large frying pan with spray light oil and fry the onions over a medium heat for a few minutes to soften. Push the onions to one side of the pan and sear the beef brisket on all sides to seal before adding the beef and onions to a slow cooker.

2. Place the carrots and mushrooms in the slow cooker along with the orange juice, red wine, garlic and ginger. Crumble in the beef stock cube and add a good pinch each of salt and pepper.

3. Finally, chop the fresh oranges in half, squeeze the juice into the slow cooker then drop the oranges in too. Set the slow cooker on high and cook for 8 hours.

4. Shred the beef brisket with two forks 45 minutes before the end of the cooking time. Spoon a little of the stew liquid into a cup and mix with the cornflour to make a thin paste. Pour the cornflour paste into the slow cooker, give everything a good stir and leave to stew for the remaining time. If there is any unwanted fat from the meat, now is the time to skim it off and discard it.

5. To make the garlic buttery potatoes, heat the oven to 190°C/170°C fan/gas 5. Place the chopped potatoes in a saucepan and cover with boiling water. Return the water to the boil and cook the potatoes for 10 minutes then drain and leave to steam in a colander for a few minutes.

6. Melt the spread in a microwave and mix in the garlic purée and chopped parsley. Place the potatoes on a large baking tray and pour over half the garlic and herb spread. Use a spoon to move the potatoes around on the tray to coat

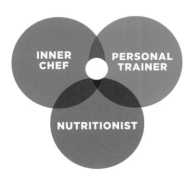

INNER CHEF
PERSONAL TRAINER
NUTRITIONIST

them with the spread. Sprinkle a good pinch of salt over the potatoes and place in the oven for 30 minutes.

7. Check the potatoes after 30 minutes, they should be golden brown and crispy on the outside. Return them to the oven if you think they need a little longer cooking time. When they are ready, take the potatoes out of the oven and pour over the remainder of the garlicky herby spread and toss to coat just before serving with the stew.

Puds

These puddings could be the most powerful weapon you possess in your nutrition plan. That's because your taste buds won't be able to tell the difference when eating these calorie-conscious alternatives. However, your leaner waistline will, as protein-packed cakes, brownies, cookies and flapjacks all serve to 'flavour' your fat loss.

CALORIES 171
PROTEIN 4g
FAT 6g
CARBS 24g
SUGARS 9g

**SERVES
9**

PLANT-BASED CHOCOLATE FUDGE CAKE

Preparation time: 10 minutes
Cooking time: 25 minutes

300ml soya milk
100ml agave syrup
1 tsp vanilla extract
100g zero-calorie granulated
    white sugar replacer
50g cocoa powder
150g self-raising flour
½ tsp baking powder
1 tsp bicarbonate of soda

FOR THE FROSTING
20g vegan chocolate
200g avocado (approximately
    1 large avocado)
100g zero-calorie powdered
    icing sugar replacer
1 tsp vanilla extract
15g cocoa powder

This dessert almost defies logic and boasts a very low-calorie content. An indulgently moist, dense, chocolate fudge cake with the creamiest chocolate frosting, it's the perfect pudding for anyone who needs their sweet tooth taming when sticking to a healthy, controlled nutrition plan.

1. Preheat the oven to 180°C/160°C fan/gas 4 and line a 20 x 20-cm square baking tin with parchment paper.

2. Either with a stand mixer or a hand-held electric mixer, whisk together the soya milk, agave syrup, vanilla extract and sweetener. Add the cocoa powder, self-raising flour, baking powder and bicarbonate of soda and whisk until fully combined. (Due to there being no oil or fat in the mixture, the batter is a little more liquidy than usual to keep the sponge moist.)

3. Pour the cake batter into the lined baking tin and place into the preheated oven for 25 minutes. You can check whether the cake is ready by poking a skewer into the centre of the cake – it should come out clean. Remove the cake from the oven and leave to cool in the tin for 10 minutes, then turn out onto a wire rack to cool completely.

4. While the chocolate fudge cake is cooling, place the chocolate in a heatproof bowl over a pan of simmering water, making sure it doesn't touch the water. Gently melt the chocolate, stirring occasionally. (Alternatively, place the bowl in a microwave and heat for no more than 6 seconds at a time, stirring each time until the chocolate has fully melted, taking care not to burn it.) Place the melted chocolate along with the remainder of the frosting ingredients in a food processor and blend until smooth.

5. Once the cake has fully cooled, use a palette knife or the back of a spoon to smooth the frosting over the top of the chocolate fudge cake, then cut into squares to serve.

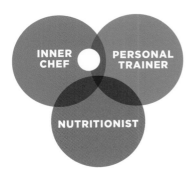

INNER CHEF PERSONAL TRAINER NUTRITIONIST

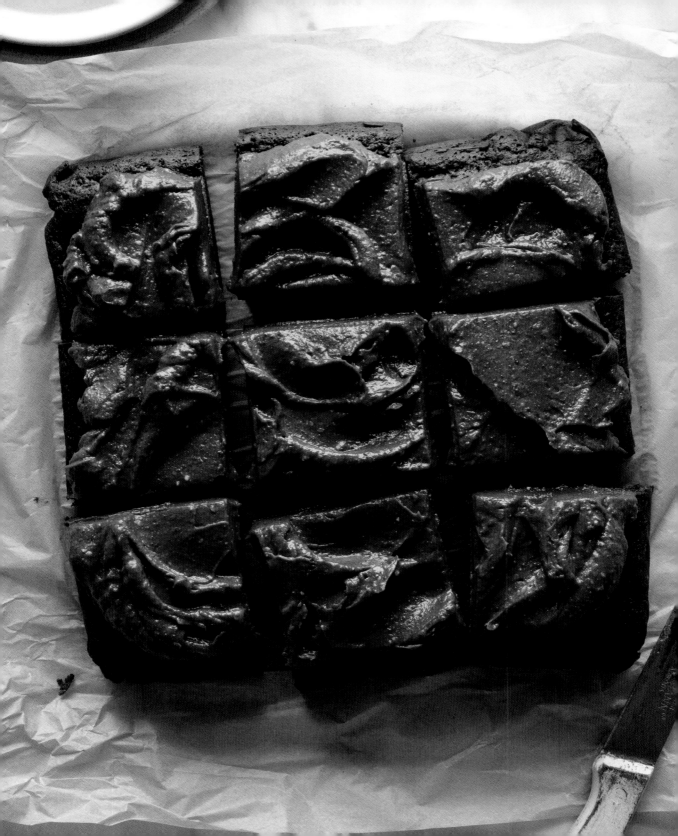

CALORIES 167
PROTEIN 6g
FAT 14g
CARBS 17g
SUGARS 3g

LEMON & BLUEBERRY PUDDING

Preparation time: 20 minutes
Cooking time: 50 minutes

3 eggs
100g zero-calorie granulated
   white sugar replacer
60g coconut oil, melted
300g 0%-fat Greek yogurt
50g Philadelphia Lightest cream
   cheese (or other low-fat
   cream cheese)
40g coconut flour
juice and zest of 2 lemons
50g fresh blueberries
zero-calorie powdered icing
   sugar replacer, for dusting
spray light oil for greasing

Presenting the lightest, fluffiest, zestiest pudding in this entire book. Made with fresh lemons and blueberries (rich in antioxidants), this recipe barely impacts on your macros (and calories). Either eat by itself or pair with a low-calorie ice cream or custard. The only thing is, it's so easy to keep going back for more of this pudding and if you live in a house like ours you could find it's all gone before you know it!

1. Preheat the oven to 170°C/150°C fan/gas 3 and grease a 20-cm round shallow pie dish with spray light oil.

2. Separate the egg yolks and whites into two clean mixing bowls. With a hand-held electric mixer, whisk the egg whites while slowly adding the sweetener. Whisk until the egg whites are thick and stiff peaks form. Set aside.

3. Add the melted coconut oil, yogurt, cream cheese, coconut flour, lemon juice and zest to the egg yolks and whisk until fully combined.

4. With a rubber spatula, gently fold the egg white mixture into the yolk mix, taking care not to knock out the air bubbles. Fold until just combined then gently fold through the blueberries.

5. Pour the mixture into the pie dish and place in the preheated oven for 50 minutes. When baked it should be firm but springy with a beautiful golden top.

6. Remove from the oven and leave to cool for 10 minutes, dust with the powdered sweetener and serve.

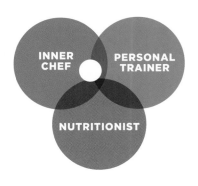

INNER CHEF
PERSONAL TRAINER
NUTRITIONIST

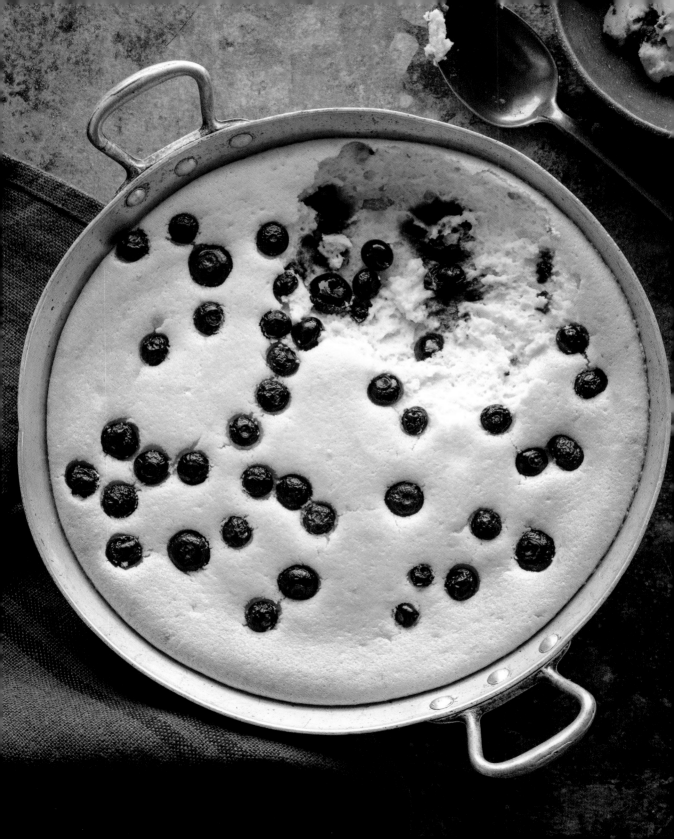

**CALORIES 209
PROTEIN 5g
FAT 6g
CARBS 31g
SUGARS 8g**

SERVES
8

RHUBARB & RASPBERRY FLAPJACK CRUMBLE

Preparation time: 10 minutes
Cooking time: 40 minutes

800g fresh rhubarb, peeled and
    roughly chopped
700g frozen raspberries
50g zero-calorie granulated
    white sugar replacer
140g porridge oats
100g plain flour
½ tsp ground cinnamon
50g zero-calorie granulated
    brown sugar replacer
100g Flora Light spread
    (or other light spread)
2 tbsp maple syrup

Recipes don't come much more wholesome and homemade than this. Presenting the Rhubarb & Raspberry Flapjack Crumble, a hybrid of a buttery oat-based flapjack top and a tart but sweet, fruity filling. A recipe that's ideal when you want something substantial, but when you're also conscious of your calories for the day. This works so well with the Vanilla Pod Ice Cream (see page 188).

1. Preheat the oven to 190°C/170°C fan/gas 5.

2. Place the rhubarb, raspberries and white sweetener into a large saucepan over a medium heat and let the fruit come to the boil. Immediately turn the heat down to a simmer and let the fruit slowly cook for 15 minutes until the rhubarb is tender.

3. In a large mixing bowl, mix together the oats, flour, cinnamon and brown sweetener. Add the spread in small pieces and lightly rub together using your fingertips to form little clusters of flapjack chunks. Do not let it form into a dough mixture.

4. Pour the fruit mixture into a large, deep pie dish or cast-iron frying pan. (We use a 24 x 4.5-cm round cast-iron frying pan.)

5. Scatter the flapjack crumble mix over the top of the fruit and drizzle the maple syrup over the crumble.

6. Place the crumble in the oven for 25 minutes or until it has turned golden brown. Serve warm with custard, or Vanilla Pod Ice Cream (see page 188), if you like.

Tip: Depending on the raspberries you're using, the fruit mixture might have quite a lot of liquid before baking. If this is the case, you can always spoon out a little of the liquid and keep it to stir through yogurt.

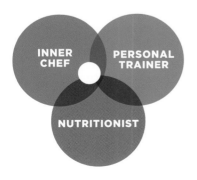

INNER CHEF · PERSONAL TRAINER · NUTRITIONIST

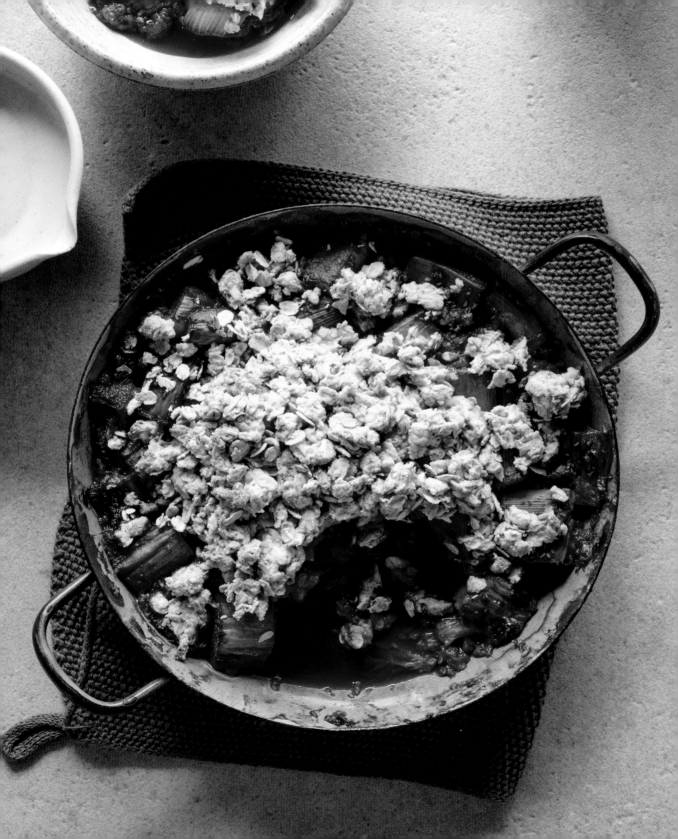

CALORIES 169
PROTEIN 12g
FAT 5g
CARBS 20g
SUGARS 6g

SERVES 9

PROTEIN ROCKY ROAD BROWNIES

Preparation time: 10 minutes
Cooking time: 15–20 minutes

400ml water
3 scoops (75g) plant-based
    chocolate protein powder
60g self-raising flour
40g cocoa powder
3 tbsp zero-calorie granulated
    white sugar replacer
50g low-fat digestive biscuits
5 Oreo biscuits
1 PhD Smart Bar cookies &
    cream flavour
20g vegan mini marshmallows
low-calorie chocolate sauce

A protein-packed chocolatey treat with all the textures for something sweet after your meal. This recipe is by far our most-baked recipe in the kitchen and even I have become a pro at making this. We'd normally pair it with a low-calorie high-protein ice cream (see page 171), so it's a PROPER PUDDING!

1. Preheat the oven to 180°C/160°C fan/gas 4 and line a 20 x 20-cm square baking tin with parchment paper.

2. In a large bowl, whisk together the water, chocolate protein powder, flour, cocoa powder and sweetener until it is a thick and smooth consistency.

3. Crush the digestives, Oreos and Smart bar into rough chunks, leaving a few pieces aside to decorate, and add the remainder to the brownie mixture. Add the marshmallows to the mix, again, holding a few back to decorate the top.

4. Place the brownie mixture into the lined baking tin and decorate the top with the remainder of the biscuits, marshmallows and Smart bar.

5. Drizzle over some liquid chocolate and bake in the preheated oven for 15–20 minutes until the brownie is evenly baked and firm to the touch.

6. Remove the brownie from the oven and leave to cool and firm up for 15 minutes before turning out onto a plate and cutting into squares. Feel free to drizzle a little more chocolate syrup on top, if you like!

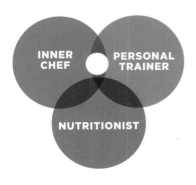

INNER CHEF
PERSONAL TRAINER
NUTRITIONIST

**CALORIES 255
PROTEIN 24g
FAT 4g
CARBS 32g
SUGARS 20g**

SERVES
4

BANANA PROTEIN ICE CREAM

Preparation time: 35 minutes
Freezing time: 6 hours

2 small bananas
2 scoops (50g) banana protein
   powder
500g 0%-fat yogurt
100ml oat milk
1 tsp xanthan gum powder
100ml Elmlea single light cream
   45% less fat

I LOVE ICE CREAM! The problem is it's traditionally made with full-fat milk, cream and plenty of sugar. Thankfully, this recipe changes all of that! It's really simple to make, low in calories and with the protein content jacked right up; perhaps the best thing about this particular alternative is that your taste buds will barely notice the difference when compared to the real thing.

1. Blitz all the ingredients together in a blender until the mixture has a thick and smooth consistency.

2. If you're using an ice cream machine, set up the bowl and mixer equipment according to the manufacturer's instructions, you may need to place the bowl in the freezer for up to 12 hours before use. Pour the ice cream mixture into the bowl and mix continuously for 30 minutes. (If you're not using an ice cream machine you can freeze the mixture for 6 hours at this stage. You might find that the ice cream is not quite as smooth as it would be when made in an ice cream machine, however, it will still taste delicious.)

3. After 30 minutes in the ice cream machine, spoon the ice cream into a freezer-safe airtight container and place in the freezer for 6 hours.

4. Remove the ice cream from the freezer 30 minutes before serving to thaw slightly for a softer scoop, if you prefer.

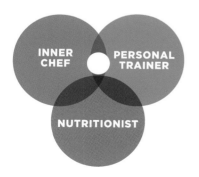

INNER CHEF

PERSONAL TRAINER

NUTRITIONIST

CALORIES 158
PROTEIN 5g
FAT 3g
CARBS 27g
SUGARS 25g

SERVES
6

MANGO FROGURT

Preparation time: 20 minutes
Freezing time: 8 hours

1kg frozen mango pieces
500g dairy-free plain yogurt
1 tbsp zero-calorie granulated
    white sugar replacer
mint sprigs and sliced
    strawberries or blueberries,
    to decorate (optional)

This recipe is essentially a cross between a yoghurt, ice cream and a fruit sorbet. It also looks (and tastes) like summer. This is because Mother Nature did a pretty awesome job when creating the refreshing, citrusy flavour of mangos and it's best not to tamper with that too much. Instead, simply invest in a blender and ice-cream maker and densely pack as much as possible into a bowl, serve, and enjoy whilst lying on the grass in the sun.

1. Remove the mango pieces from the freezer 30 minutes before using, to thaw a little.

2. Place the mango pieces in a blender along with the yogurt and sweetener and blitz until the mixture has a thick and smooth consistency. (You may need to scrape down the sides of the blender a few times.)

3. The sorbet should now be thick enough to serve immediately, if you wish. If you want an even firmer texture you can churn the mixture in an ice cream machine for 15–20 minutes then pour it into a freezer-safe airtight container and place in the freezer for 8 hours. (If you're not using an ice cream machine you can freeze the mixture for 8 hours at this stage. You might find that the frogurt is not quite as aerated and smooth as it would be when made in an ice cream machine, however, it will still taste delicious.)

4. Serve the sorbet in a small bowl or glass and decorate with a sprig of fresh mint, slices of fresh strawberry or a few blueberries, if you like.

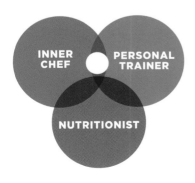

INNER CHEF

PERSONAL TRAINER

NUTRITIONIST

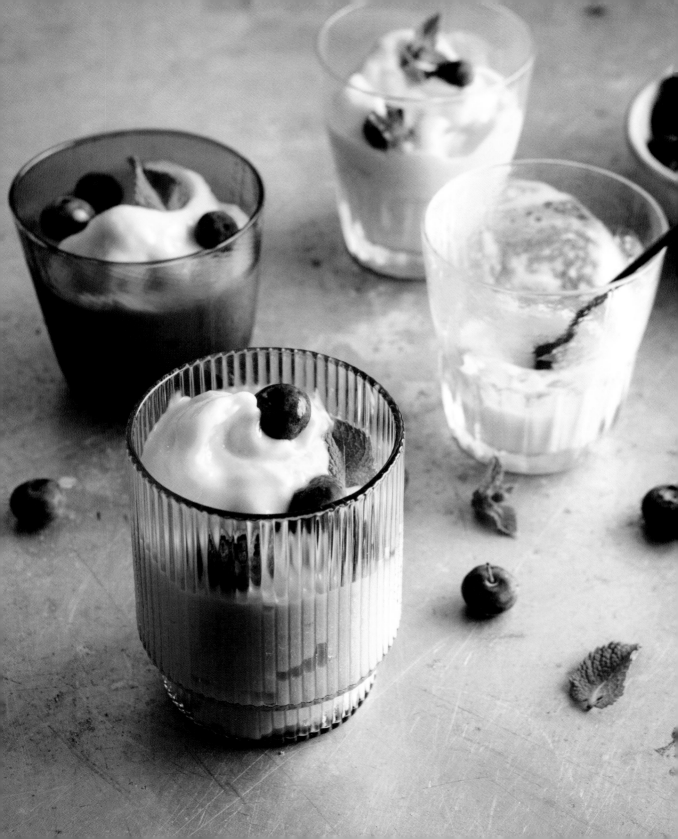

SERVES 10

CARROT CAKE

Preparation time: 20 minutes
Cooking time: 25–30 minutes

100g walnuts, chopped
300g self-raising flour
3 eggs
60g apple sauce
100g zero-calorie brown sugar replacer
150g zero-calorie granulated white sugar replacer
150ml pineapple juice
120ml buttermilk
1 tsp vanilla extract
2 tsp mixed spice
1 tsp ground ginger
2 tsp ground cinnamon
2 tsp baking powder
2 tsp bicarbonate of soda
200g carrots, grated
50g tinned pineapple, chopped into small chunks
spray light oil for greasing

FOR THE CREAM CHEESE TOPPING
180g Philadelphia Lightest cream cheese (or other low-fat cream cheese)
1 tbsp lemon juice
200g zero-calorie powdered icing sugar replacer

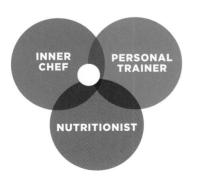

INNER CHEF

PERSONAL TRAINER

NUTRITIONIST

In 2016, we visited the island of Nevis in the Caribbean where I completed a 'treeathlon' (an Olympic-distance triathlon carrying a 100-lb tree) for charity. Not only was the event a huge success, we also found the world's greatest carrot cake and became obsessed with creating our own healthy version. Conventional carrot cake recipes are known for using a lot of oil and sugar, so the challenge was to halve the calories but keep the taste, texture and flavour. After many, many trials it worked! Containing only 252 calories per slice. It's so incredibly moist and loaded with tonnes of pineapple and earthy spices.

1. Preheat the oven to 170°C/150°C fan/gas 3 and line the bases and grease the sides of two 20-cm round baking tins.

2. Mix 75g of the chopped walnuts with 1 tablespoon of the flour in a small bowl and set aside. This will help prevent the walnuts from sinking to the bottom of the cake batter.

3. With a hand-held electric mixer, whisk together the eggs, apple sauce, brown and granulated sweeteners, pineapple juice, buttermilk and vanilla extract.

4. Whisk all of the dry ingredients into the wet mixture until it forms a thick cake batter. Fold the grated carrot and pineapple chunks into the cake batter with a rubber spatula and finally fold in the floured walnuts.

5. Divide the mixture between the two cake tins and bake in the preheated oven for 25–30 minutes until a skewer inserted into the middle of the cake comes out clean.

6. Remove the cakes from the oven and leave to cool in the tins for 10 minutes, then turn out onto wire racks to cool completely.

7. To make the cream cheese frosting, either with a stand mixer or a hand-held electric mixer, whisk together the cream cheese, lemon juice and powdered sweetener until smooth and creamy.

8. If your cakes are a little domed, take a bread knife and cut the dome horizontally to level off the cake on one of the sponges. The cut cake will be your bottom layer. Spread half the frosting onto the base layer of cake then stack the second sponge on top. Spread the remainder of the frosting evenly over the top of the cake and sprinkle over the remaining chopped walnuts.

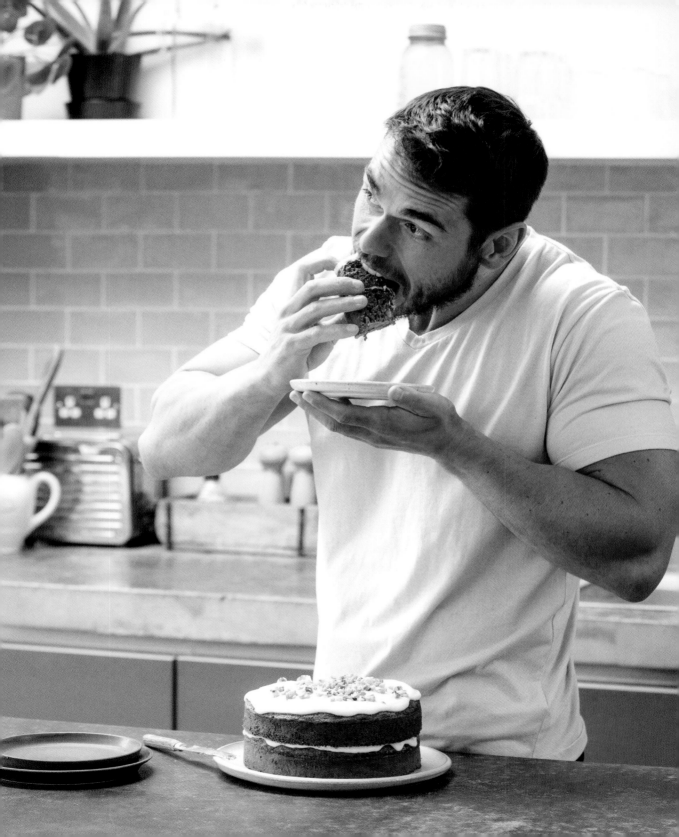

CALORIES 82
PROTEIN 5g
FAT 2g
CARBS 12g
SUGARS 6g

Preparation time: 10 minutes
Cooking time: 12–15 minutes

400g soya yogurt
1 tsp vanilla extract
250g self-raising flour
1 tsp bicarbonate of soda
2 tsp baking powder
100g zero-calorie granulated
    white sugar replacer
144ml vegan whippable cream
120g reduced-sugar jam,
    traditionally strawberry is
    used, but raspberry also
    works well
zero-calorie powdered icing
    sugar replacer, for dusting

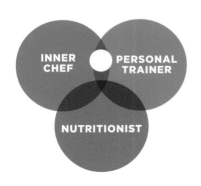

INNER CHEF
PERSONAL TRAINER
NUTRITIONIST

VEGAN VICTORIA SPONGE TOPS

Presenting the most quintessentially British sweet treat ever created; the Victoria Sponge Cake. Soft, fluffy, light and layered with jam, the issue is often the sugar and calorie content, which is why Hester worked tirelessly to create our own version that's low in calories and easily fits into your macro requirements for the day.

1. Preheat the oven to 180°C/160°C fan/gas 4 and line a 12-hole muffin tin with cupcake cases.

2. Mix the soya yogurt and vanilla extract together in one bowl and mix all the dry ingredients together in another.

3. With a hand-held electric mixer, gradually incorporate the dry mix into the wet mixture until fully combined. Scrape down the sides of the bowl to ensure no excess flour is stuck to the bottom of the bowl and mix for a few more seconds on high speed.

4. Pour a quarter of the mixture into a piping bag and set aside while you split the remainder of the mix between the 12 cupcake cases.

5. Line a baking sheet with some parchment paper and use the remaining mixture in the piping bag to pipe 12 rounds of batter about 3cm wide to make the tops for your cakes.

6. Place the cupcakes into the preheated oven and bake for 12–15 minutes until risen and golden brown. Remove from the oven and leave on a wire rack to cool completely. The piped rounds for the tops won't take as long to bake, so wait until the cupcakes are cooked then bake them for 5–6 minutes, while the cupcakes cool. The tops are ready when they have turned golden brown (keep a close eye on them as they can easily burn).

7. Pour the vegan cream into a mixing bowl and whisk with a hand-held electric mixer until the cream has stiff peaks.

8. Spoon a small amount of jam and a small amount of whipped cream onto each cupcake, then gently place a sponge top on the jam and whipped cream. Finish with a little dusting of powdered sweetener before serving.

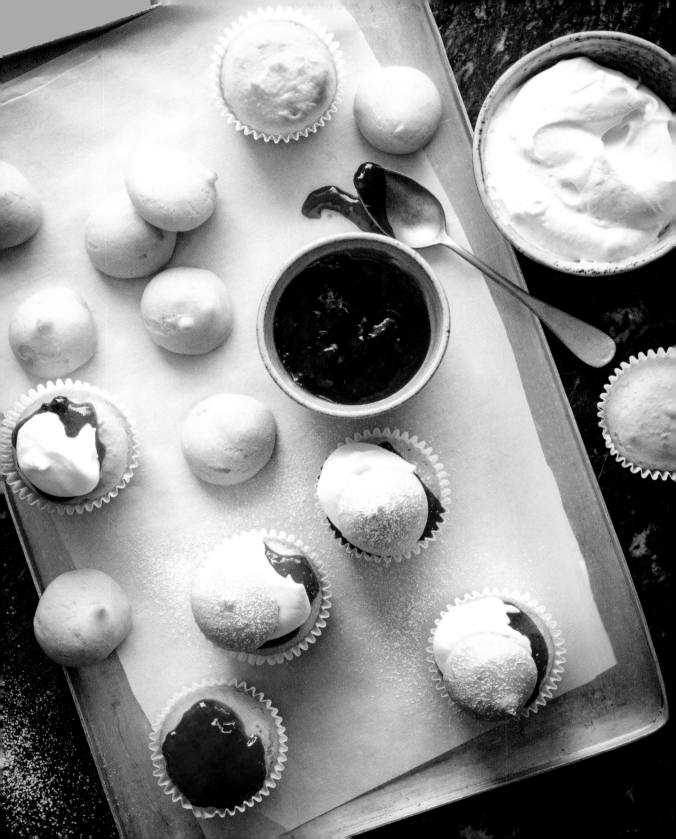

CALORIES 139
PROTEIN 4g
FAT 7g
CARBS 14g
SUGARS 0.9g

LEMON DRIZZLE TRAYBAKE

Preparation time: 15 minutes
Cooking time: 25 minutes

200g zero-calorie granulated
    white sugar replacer
225g Flora Light spread (or
    other light spread)
3 eggs
225g self-raising flour
1 tsp baking powder
juice and zest of 2 lemons

FOR THE LEMON SOAK
6 tbsp lemon juice
1 tbsp zero-calorie granulated
    white sugar replacer

FOR THE GLAZE
150g zero-calorie powdered
    icing sugar replacer
4–5 tbsp lemon juice
sprinkles (optional)

Every kitchen cupboard should come equipped with the ingredients for this recipe. Light and packed with a sweet, citrus flavour, it's easy to make and ideal when you want something homemade that will stop you reaching for those unhealthy alternative snacks. Glazed with a no-sugar icing alternative, it can be stored in an airtight container like a secret weapon in weight loss, as this recipe should last you the week!

1. Preheat the oven to 180°C/160°C fan/gas 4 and line a 26 x 20-cm rectangular baking tin with parchment paper.

2. Using a stand mixer or hand-held electric mixer, whisk together the sweetener and spread until light and fluffy.

3. One by one, whisk in the eggs then add the flour and baking powder and mix again before finally adding the lemon juice and zest. Mix once more to make sure all the ingredients are combined.

4. Pour the batter into the lined baking tin and place in the preheated oven for 25 minutes, until a skewer inserted into the middle of the cake comes out clean.

5. While the cake is baking, make the lemon soak by mixing the lemon juice and granulated sweetener in a small saucepan over a low heat until the sweetener has dissolved.

6. As soon as you remove the cake from the oven, prick it all over with a skewer and brush the lemon soak over the entire surface of the sponge, allowing it to seep in.

7. Finally, mix together the powdered sweetener and lemon juice in a small bowl to make the glaze. Pour the glaze on top of the cooled traybake and add a few sprinkles for a pop of colour, if you like. This bit isn't necessary but it's fun to make it look a little prettier!

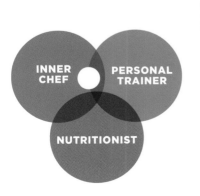

INNER CHEF   PERSONAL TRAINER

NUTRITIONIST

CALORIES 258
PROTEIN 8g
FAT 6g
CARBS 42g
SUGARS 11g

SERVES 4

CINNAMON & GINGER RICE PROTEIN PUDDING POTS

Preparation time: 10 minutes
Cooking time: 1 hour 10 minutes

100g pudding rice
700ml oat milk
100ml Elmlea single light cream 45% less fat
60g zero-calorie granulated white sugar replacer
1 tsp vanilla bean paste
2 tsp ground cinnamon
1 tsp ground ginger
50g raisins
1 scoop (25g) vanilla protein powder

I cannot express how much I love rice pudding. It basically tastes like my childhood, since my mum makes the best homemade rice pudding (from scratch) and it's the sweetest, creamiest, baked rice pudding you've ever seen. But when trying to keep my bodyweight down, I need a lower-calorie version, which is why we created the Cinnamon & Ginger Rice Protein Pudding Pots. For me, they're the perfect autumn dessert and can be eaten hot or cold.

1. Preheat the oven to 150°C/130°C fan/gas 2.

2. Wash and drain the rice. Pour all the ingredients, apart from the raisins, into a deep-sided baking dish about 20cm wide and gently whisk together with a balloon whisk. Place the baking dish in the oven and bake for 40 minutes.

3. After 40 minutes, remove the rice pudding from the oven. If a skin has formed on the surface, remove it and give the rice pudding a good stir. Next, stir in the raisins and place back in the oven for a further 30 minutes.

4. At the end of the cooking time the pudding will be baked through and there should be a delicious layer of golden skin on top of the creamiest rice pudding.

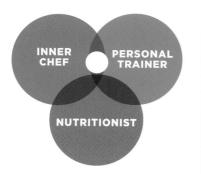

INNER CHEF

PERSONAL TRAINER

NUTRITIONIST

CALORIES 275
PROTEIN 10g
FAT 11g
CARBS 32g
SUGARS 14g

SERVES
5

Preparation time: 2 hours
Cooking time: 40 minutes

3 small ripe bananas, peeled
50g tahini
100g fat-free yogurt
1 tbsp vanilla extract
1 large egg
60g plain flour
1 tsp bicarbonate of soda
50g zero-calorie granulated
 white sugar replacer
50g low-calorie brown sugar
 replacer
25g cocoa powder
50g dark chocolate chips
spray light oil for greasing

BANANA & CHOCOLATE PUDDING

The sole purpose of this recipe is to satisfy your sweet cravings (and to keep your inner chef and inner personal trainer happy). Think of it as a chocolate-covered secret weapon you have in your toolbox when dieting – all because you won't find a dessert that packs as much flavour, taste, texture and indulgence into 275 calories per slice – keeping your taste buds satisfied and your body fat in check. It's virtually indistinguishable from even its most calorie-dense rivals and perfect for that weekend dessert when family and friends visit for Sunday dinner. They will never notice the difference!

1. Preheat the oven to 180°C/160°C fan/gas 4 and grease a 20 x 20 x 5-cm square, baking dish (or 23-cm round, deep dish) with spray light oil.

2. Use a hand-held electric mixer or stand mixer to mash up the peeled ripe bananas then add in the tahini, yogurt and vanilla extract and mix on a slow speed until fully combined. Add the egg and whisk again.

3. In a separate bowl, mix together the flour, bicarbonate of soda, both sweeteners and cocoa powder then gradually whisk the dry mixture into the wet mixture, adding a few spoonfuls at a time. Finally, stir through the dark chocolate chips.

4. Pour the pudding mixture into the greased baking dish and bake in the preheated oven for 40 minutes. The pudding should look baked on top but with a gooey centre.

5. Remove from the oven and rest for 10 minutes to firm up a bit before serving.

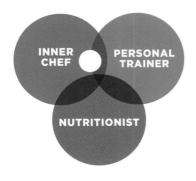

INNER CHEF

PERSONAL TRAINER

NUTRITIONIST

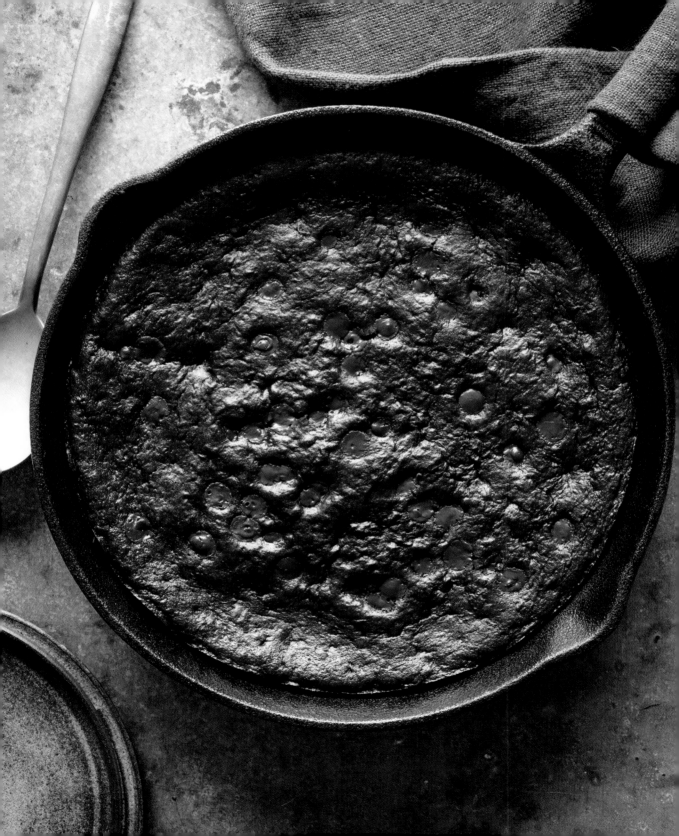

CALORIES 281
PROTEIN 14g
FAT 4g
CARBS 45g
SUGARS 30g

SERVES
4

STICKY TOFFEE PROTEIN PUDDING

Preparation time: 20 minutes
Cooking time: 40 minutes

130g dried pitted dates (medjool dates are preferable but not essential)
200ml strong black tea (use 2 tea bags)
2 eggs, yolks and whites separated
2 scoops (50g) salted caramel or vanilla protein powder
65g fine plain wholemeal flour
1 tsp baking powder
30g maple syrup for the base of the pudding pot, plus 30g for drizzling, to serve
spray light oil for greasing

Sticky toffee pudding is a fan favourite with many, but this sticky toffee protein pudding is a fan favourite with everyone. Containing the same rich, caramel flavour (yet with no added sugar) you would barely be able to notice that it's a much healthier alternative. A deliciously moist, cakey texture, drenched with a sweet maple syrup to top it off. This one is honestly hard to believe – there are only 281 calories per portion, with 14g of protein to add to your macros!

1. Preheat the oven to 170°C/150°C fan/gas 3.

2. Place the dates in a saucepan and add the black tea. Place the pan over a medium heat and let the dates soften a little for a few minutes. Place the date and tea mixture into a blender and blitz until a smooth paste forms.

3. Using a hand-held electric mixer, whisk the two egg whites in a clean mixing bowl until they become glossy and stiff peaks form, then set aside.

4. In a separate bowl, mix together the protein powder, egg yolks, flour, baking powder and date paste until a smooth and thick batter forms.

5. Use a silicon spatula to gently fold half the whipped egg whites into the sponge batter mix, taking care not to knock the air bubbles out of the mixture. Repeat with the remainder of the whipped egg whites.

6. Grease four individual pudding moulds with spray light oil. Spoon half a tablespoon of maple syrup into the bottom of each one then split the cake mixture evenly between them. Wrap a piece of aluminium foil around the top of each pudding mould and place in a deep oven dish.

7. Pour boiling water into the oven dish until it reaches halfway up the pudding moulds then place in the oven for 40 minutes.

8. Once baked, you can immediately tip over your pudding pots into a bowl and drizzle another ½ tablespoon of maple syrup for the sponge to soak up the sweet rich flavours.

9. Serve with a scoop of homemade Vanilla Pod Ice Cream (see page 190) or a reduced-fat single cream.

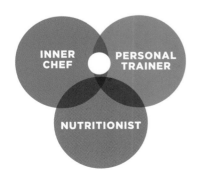

INNER CHEF
PERSONAL TRAINER
NUTRITIONIST

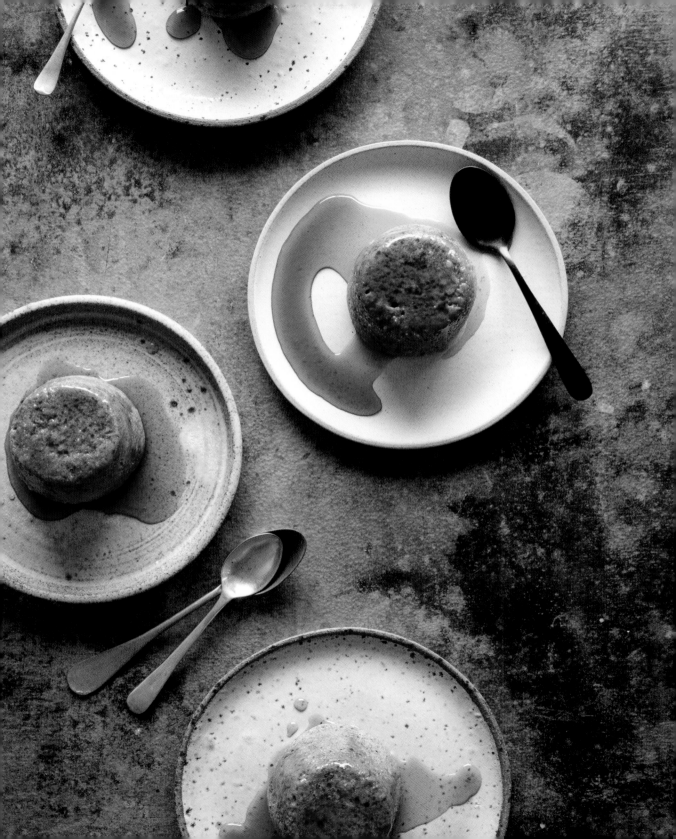

CALORIES 281
PROTEIN 6g
FAT 5g
CARBS 63g
SUGARS 27g

SERVES 8

CHERRY BAKEWELL SPONGE PUDDING

Preparation time: 20 minutes
Cooking time: 20 minutes

80ml agave syrup
250ml soya milk
2 tsp almond extract
100g zero-calorie granulated white sugar replacer
300g self-raising flour
1 tsp baking powder
25g ground almonds
20g almond flakes

FOR THE FILLING
1kg frozen pitted cherries
50g black cherry jam, use a reduced-sugar variety if you prefer
2 tbsp zero-calorie granulated white sugar replacer

Our Cherry Bakewell Sponge Pudding took everyone's favourite recipe and nutritionally reformulated it into a lighter alternative, so your taste buds love it as much as your tummy. Containing a light, moist, almond sponge lying on top of a bed of juicy sweet cherries, it's then decorated with toasted almond flakes and is best served with ice cream, custard or (in my case) both!

1. Preheat the oven to 180°C/160°C fan/gas 4.

2. Make the filling by placing the frozen cherries, black cherry jam and sweetener into a large saucepan over a medium heat. Leave to simmer for about 20 minutes until the cherries have softened and the juice from them has reduced by half.

3. While the cherries are cooking, make the almond cake batter by mixing the wet ingredients together in a mixing bowl. Whisk in all the dry ingredients until fully combined. Scrape down the sides of the bowl to make sure all the ingredients are mixed in and not stuck to the bottom of the bowl, then whisk for a further few seconds.

4. Pour the cherry filling into a 23cm x 5-cm deep round, or 20 x 20 x 5-cm deep square baking dish and spread it out evenly, then gently spoon the almond cake batter on top, smoothing it over the cherries. Sprinkle the almond flakes on top of the cake batter and place into the preheated oven for 20 minutes or until the top of the sponge is a light golden colour with a springy but firm texture.

5. Remove from the oven and rest for 5–10 minutes before serving.

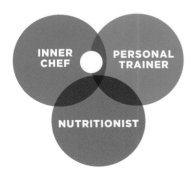

INNER CHEF · PERSONAL TRAINER · NUTRITIONIST

**CALORIES 294
PROTEIN 14g
FAT 10g
CARBS 35g
SUGARS 18g**

GIANT PROTEIN SKILLET COOKIE

SERVES 6

Preparation time: 20 minutes
Cooking time: 30–35 minutes

2 x 400g tins chickpeas,
   drained and rinsed
100g 0%-fat yogurt
2 tsp vanilla extract
50g almond butter
50g maple syrup
50g soft brown sugar
30g self-raising flour
1 scoop (25g) vanilla protein
   powder
½ tsp bicarbonate of soda
2 tsp baking powder
50g extra dark chocolate
   chunks
butter flavour spray light oil
   for greasing

In my opinion, this is how every cookie should be made and served. Extra-large and enriched with protein, this is a much healthier alternative to a full-on, sugar-loaded, cookie dough skillet, but it is just as gooey and chewy on the inside and crispy and crunchy on the outside. As with so many puddings, the Vanilla Pod Ice Cream (see page 188) makes a perfect pairing.

1. Preheat the oven to 170°C/150°C fan/gas 3 and grease a 23-cm cast-iron pan with the spray light oil.

2. Add the chickpeas, yogurt, vanilla extract, almond butter, maple syrup and brown sugar to a blender and blitz until the mixture becomes a smooth and thick consistency. Pour into a mixing bowl then add the flour, protein powder, bicarbonate of soda, baking powder and three-quarters of the chocolate chips, stirring everything together until combined.

3. Pour the chocolate chip cookie mixture into the cast-iron pan and sprinkle the rest of the chocolate chips on top.

4. Place the giant cookie in the oven for 30–35 minutes. The cookie dough should be baked and golden on the outside with a softer, gooey centre. If the mixture is still a little runny in the centre, leave it in the oven for a further few minutes.

5. Remove from the oven and rest in the pan for 10–15 minutes before serving.

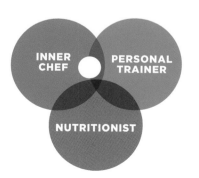

INNER CHEF
PERSONAL TRAINER
NUTRITIONIST

SERVES
12

ORANGE & ALMOND CAKE

Preparation time: 1 hour
    40 minutes
Cooking time: 40–45 minutes

2 whole oranges
225g zero-calorie granulated
    white sugar replacer
4 eggs
1 tsp almond extract
240g ground almonds
1 tsp baking powder
25g flaked almonds

Whenever we are in London, we go on a huge food pilgrimage and attack our favourite bakeries armed with a spoon, fork and napkin. But one of them in particular has the most amazing Orange and Almond Cake. Every time we walk in it's there, sat on the top of the counter with a crusty edge and toasted flaked almond top, and a moist, melt-in-the-middle, sweet almond and orangey centre. Unfortunately, it also boasts a pretty impressive calorie count, which is not ideal when you're training to keep your bodyweight in check. Fortunately, Hester is a genius and was able to tweak and tailor the recipe to bring the fat content and calorie count way down, so now we can enjoy a slice with a dollop of homemade Protein Vanilla Pod Ice Cream – check out the recipe on page 188.

1. Cut the ends off both the oranges and place them in a saucepan of boiling water. Simmer for 1 hour 30 minutes, topping up the water every so often to make sure the oranges remain completely submerged.

2. Remove the oranges from the pan, drain them and set aside to cool. Preheat the oven to 170°C/150°C fan/gas 3 and line a 23-cm round baking tin with parchment paper.

3. Once the oranges have cooled, chop them into rough chunks, place in a blender and blitz to a purée.

4. With a stand mixer or hand-held electric mixer, whisk together the sweetener, eggs and almond extract. Add the ground almonds, baking powder and orange purée and mix together until fully combined.

6. Pour the cake batter into the lined baking tin and sprinkle the flaked almonds evenly over the top. Place in the preheated oven for 40–45 minutes or until a skewer inserted into the centre of the cake comes out clean. The cake will be a lovely golden brown colour.

7. Remove the cake from the oven and leave to cool in the tin for 20 minutes before tucking in.

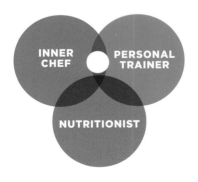

INNER CHEF
PERSONAL TRAINER
NUTRITIONIST

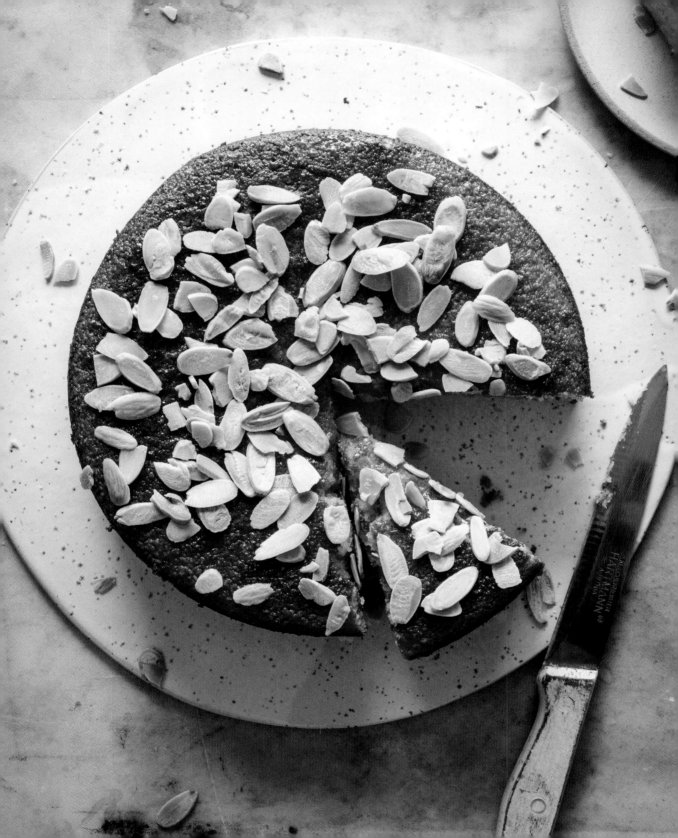

SERVES
4

VANILLA POD ICE CREAM

Preparation time: 35 minutes
Freezing time: 6 hours

3 scoops (75g) vanilla
   protein powder
500g 0%-fat yogurt
200ml Elmlea single light cream
   45% less fat
100ml oat milk
1 tsp xanthan gum powder
1 tsp vanilla bean paste
1 tsp vanilla extract

This low-calorie, high-protein ice cream is a real staple in our house. We usually have this on a weekday after our tea for something sweet with a light hot chocolate. Equally, this recipe pairs so well with pretty much all the baked desserts in this book – our favourites being the Cherry Bakewell Cake and the Banana & Chocolate Pudding.

1. Blitz all the ingredients together in a blender until the mixture has a thick and smooth consistency.

2. If you're using an ice cream machine, set up the bowl and mixer equipment according to the manufacturer's instructions, you may need to place the bowl in the freezer for up to 12 hours before use. Pour the ice cream mixture into the bowl and mix continuously for 30 minutes. (If you're not using an ice cream machine you can freeze the mixture for 6 hours at this stage. You might find that the ice cream is not quite as smooth as it would be when made in an ice cream machine, however, it will still taste delicious.)

3. After 30 minutes in the ice cream machine, spoon the ice cream into a freezer-safe airtight container and place in the freezer for 6 hours.

4. Remove the ice cream from the freezer 30 minutes before serving to thaw slightly for a softer scoop, if you prefer.

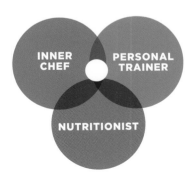

INNER CHEF

PERSONAL TRAINER

NUTRITIONIST

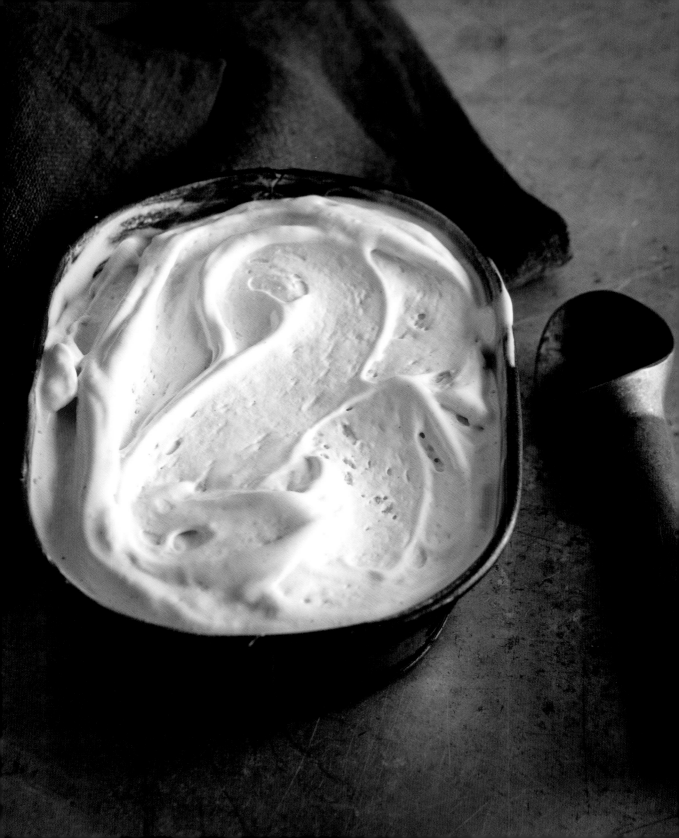

Cheesecake Game

When it comes to dessert, the cheesecake reigns supreme. This is why it only made logical sense to devote an entire section to it in all its forms. From the very best healthy banoffee recipe you'll ever taste to our newest caramelised biscuit-base creation, each is naturally high in protein and can be nutritionally re-engineered to support any dietary goal.

CALORIES 208
PROTEIN 12g
FAT 8g
CARBS 32g
SUGAR 14g

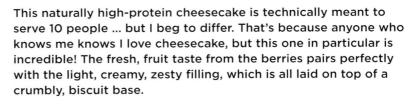

SERVES
10

NO-BAKE LEMON & BLUEBERRY CHEESECAKE

Preparation time: 20 minutes
Setting time: 24 hours

FOR THE BASE
23 Lotus Biscoff biscuits
30g coconut oil

FOR THE FILLING
4 gelatine sheets
400g Philadelphia Lightest
   cream cheese (or other
   low-fat cream cheese)
500g fat-free quark
100g zero-calorie granulated
   white sugar replacer
150ml lemon juice
200g blueberries, fresh or
   frozen

TO DECORATE
50g fresh blueberries
½ tbsp lemon zest
zero-calorie powdered icing
   sugar replacer, for dusting

This naturally high-protein cheesecake is technically meant to serve 10 people ... but I beg to differ. That's because anyone who knows me knows I love cheesecake, but this one in particular is incredible! The fresh, fruit taste from the berries pairs perfectly with the light, creamy, zesty filling, which is all laid on top of a crumbly, biscuit base.

1. Place the biscuits in a heavy-duty freezer or sandwich bag and crush with a rolling pin until you have fine crumbs. Melt the coconut oil in the microwave in 7-second intervals until melted. Pour the crushed biscuits and the coconut oil into a bowl and mix together until the crumbs are fully coated in the oil.

2. Press the oily crumbs into a lined 23-cm round springform cake tin and use your hands to press the crumbs firmly and evenly into the base. Place in the fridge for 40 minutes to firm up.

3. Place the gelatine sheets in a bowl of cold water and set aside to soak for 5 minutes to soften.

4. To make the filling, whisk together the cream cheese, quark and sweetener in a large bowl until fully combined.

5. Heat the lemon juice in a small saucepan until it's just too hot to dip your finger into, then take off the heat. Squeeze the excess water from the gelatine sheets and place in the hot lemon juice, stirring the mixture for a few seconds until the gelatine dissolves.

6. Pour the lemon juice with gelatine straight into the cheesecake mix and whisk together immediately (otherwise the gelatine will go stringy if cooled and left too long before mixing). Finally, fold in the blueberries with a rubber spatula.

7. Pour the cheesecake mixture onto the chilled biscuit base, gently tap the tin on the work surface a few times to remove any big air bubbles and place in the fridge to set for 24 hours.

8. Once the cheesecake is set, remove it from the tin by carefully running a knife around the edge of the cheesecake before undoing the clasp on the side of the tin. Gently lift the tin away and very carefully slide the cheesecake onto a serving plate. Decorate with the fresh blueberries, lemon zest and a dusting of icing sugar replacer.

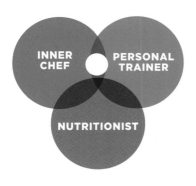

INNER CHEF
PERSONAL TRAINER
NUTRITIONIST

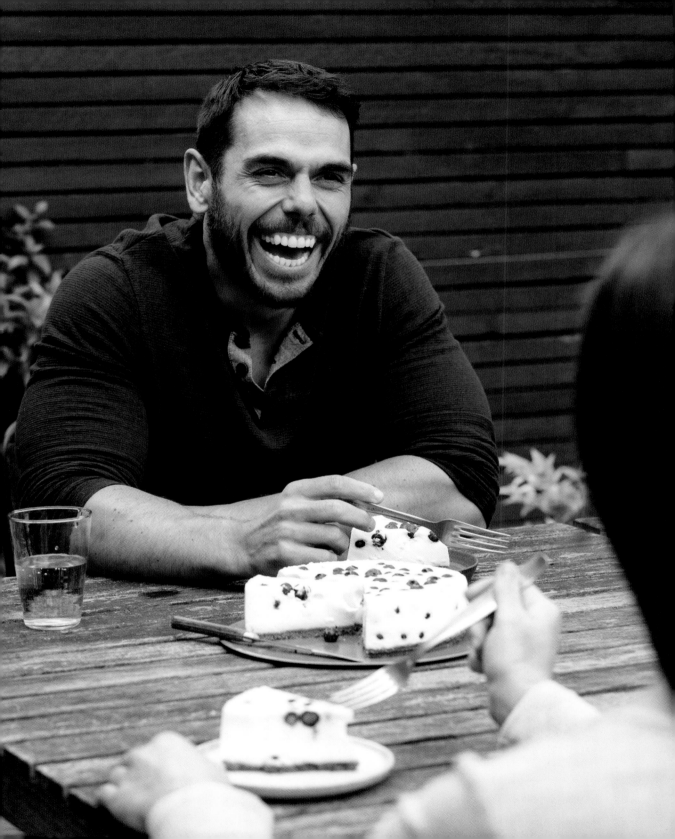

CALORIES 349
PROTEIN 13.3g
FAT 9.5g
CARBS 34.7g
SUGAR 18.5g

SERVES 10

Preparation time: 25 minutes
Cooking time: 1 hour 5 minutes

FOR THE BASE
18 digestive biscuits
30g Flora Light spread (or
    other light spread)

FOR THE FILLING
50g milk chocolate
100g zero-calorie granulated
    white sugar replacer
3 eggs
500g quark
440g Philadelphia Lightest
    cream cheese (or other
    low-fat cream cheese)
1 tsp vanilla extract
40g cocoa powder

TO DECORATE
3 crème eggs, halved
30g milk chocolate, melted
16 mini eggs

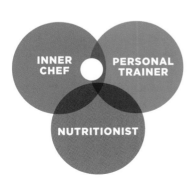

MINI EGG CHOCOLATE BAKED CHEESECAKE

We celebrate Easter a little differently in our house and put our chocolate eggs on top of a protein-enriched cheesecake. What's even better is it's lower in calories than an ordinary cheesecake, but still delivers a rich, creamy, cocoa topping on top of a moreish biscuit base.

1. Preheat the oven to 170°C/150°C fan/gas 3. Place the digestive biscuits in a heavy-duty freezer or sandwich bag and crush with a rolling pin until you have fine crumbs.

2. Melt the spread in the microwave for a few seconds, then stir into the biscuit crumbs in a small mixing bowl.

3. Tip the crumbs into a 22-cm round springform cake tin and use your hands to press them firmly and evenly into the base of the tin. Bake in the oven for 15 minutes, then set aside to cool.

4. Place the chocolate in a heatproof bowl over a pan of simmering water, making sure it doesn't touch the water. Gently melt the chocolate, stirring occasionally. (Alternatively, place the bowl in a microwave and heat for no more than 6 seconds at a time, stirring each time until the chocolate has fully melted, taking care not to burn it.)

5. Using a hand-held electric mixer, whisk together the sweetener and eggs in a large mixing bowl. Beat the mixture for a few minutes until light and fluffy then add the quark, cream cheese and vanilla extract and whisk until fully combined. Add the cocoa powder and melted chocolate and mix once more.

6. Pour the filling over the biscuit base and bake for 50 minutes. It should be firm to the touch and have risen like a soufflé. If you gently jiggle it it should only wobble very slightly in the middle.

7. Turn the oven off, open the door and place the halved crème eggs on top of the cheesecake. Leave the cheesecake to cool in the oven with the door ajar.

8. Let the cheesecake cool down fully (this could take a couple of hours) then remove from the tin and place on serving plate. Finally, drizzle over the melted chocolate and scatter the mini eggs over the top for a pop of colour.

CALORIES 281
PROTEIN 20g
FAT 14g
CARBS 20g
SUGAR 17g

SERVES
12

REESE'S PEANUT BUTTER CUP & CHOCOLATE MINI CHEESECAKES

Preparation time: 30 minutes
Cooking time: 20 minutes

FOR THE BASE
150g smooth peanut butter
50g light agave syrup
4 scoops (100g) vanilla protein powder
100ml soya milk

FOR THE FILLING
100g (about 3 large) egg whites
150g Philadelphia Lightest cream cheese (or other low-fat cream cheese)
200g 0%-fat yogurt
2 scoops (50g) chocolate protein powder
1 tbsp smooth peanut butter
1 tbsp light agave syrup

TO DECORATE
25g dark chocolate
2 tbsp smooth peanut butter
12 Reese's Peanut Butter Cups

Peanut butter has to be one of the most popular ingredients to use in heathier baking and everybody, including us, is obsessed with it! These mini baked cheesecakes are packed with protein but also give that indulgent hit of milk chocolate combined with an earthy peanut-butter flavour. A healthier alternative cheesecake that will fit into your macros as either a protein snack or mini dessert.

1. Preheat the oven to 150°C/130°C fan/gas 2.

2. To make the peanut cookie base, mix together the peanut butter, agave syrup, vanilla protein powder and soya milk to make a cookie dough type mix. Split the cookie dough between a 12-cavity mini cheesecake tin with removable bases then pop the tin in the fridge while you make the filling.

3. Using a hand-held electric mixer, whisk the egg whites in a clean mixing bowl until they become glossy and stiff peaks form, then set aside.

4. In a separate mixing bowl, mix together the cream cheese, yogurt, chocolate protein powder, peanut butter and agave syrup.

5. Use a silicone spatula to gently fold half the whipped egg whites into the cheesecake mix, taking care not to knock out the air bubbles. Repeat with the remaining whipped egg whites.

6. Spoon the cheesecake mixture on top of the 12 peanut cookie bases and place in the oven for 20 minutes.

7. Remove from the oven and leave the cheesecakes to cool in the tin for 5 minutes, then very carefully pop them out of the tin and place on a cooling rack to cool completely.

8. Place the chocolate and peanut butter in a heatproof bowl over a pan of simmering water, making sure it doesn't touch the water. Gently melt the chocolate and peanut butter, stirring occasionally. (Alternatively, place the bowl in a microwave and heat for no more than 6 seconds at a time, stirring each time until the chocolate and peanut butter has fully melted, taking care not to burn it.) Use a teaspoon to drizzle the melted chocolate and peanut butter on top of the cheesecakes and finally add a Peanut Butter Cup on top to decorate.

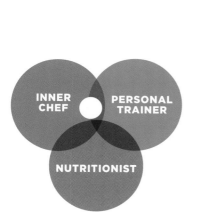

INNER CHEF

PERSONAL TRAINER

NUTRITIONIST

CALORIES 347
PROTEIN 1.5g
FAT 21.0g
CARBS 32.1g
SUGAR 10.3g

SERVES
10

VEGAN OREO CHEESECAKE

Preparation time: 30 minutes
Cooking time: 15 minutes
Setting time: 24 hours

FOR THE BASE
21 Oreos
30g Flora Light spread
(or other light spread)

FOR THE FILLING
6 Oreos
750g Violife Creamy Original
soft cheese
100g zero-calorie granulated
white sugar replacer
250g zero-calorie powdered
icing sugar replacer
1 tsp vanilla extract

TO DECORATE
1 Oreo
25g vegan chocolate

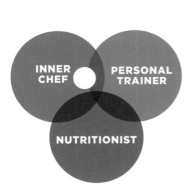

Presenting a contender for the King of Cheesecakes! This is for anyone wanting a great-tasting dessert but without the calorific content that a normal full-fat cheesecake would provide. It's also so easy to make. Made with an Oreo biscuit base, a cookies 'n' cream biscuit-flavoured cream cheese filling, drizzled with melted dark chocolate and decorated with Oreo crumb. This cheesecake is vegan so doesn't contain any gelatine, which means it will be a little softer than a regular set cheesecake. However, it still cuts into beautiful clean slices. See photo on the next page.

1. Preheat the oven to 180°C/160°C fan/gas 4 and line the base of a 23-cm round springform cake tin with parchment paper.

2. Take the 21 base Oreos, separate the biscuit from the filling and place the filling into a small bowl.

3. Take the separated biscuits, place them in a heavy-duty freezer or sandwich bag and crush with a rolling pin until you have fine crumbs. Melt the spread in the microwave for approximately 10 seconds or until melted. Pour the crushed biscuits and the melted spread into a bowl and mix together until the crumbs are fully coated in the spread.

4. Place the biscuit base mixture into the lined tin and use your hands to press the crumbs firmly and evenly into the base of the tin. Place in the preheated oven for 15 minutes then remove and set aside on a wire rack to cool completely.

5. To make the cream cheese filling, take the 6 Oreos and, again, separate the biscuits from the filling. Add in the filling from the single Oreo you have set aside to decorate the cheesecake. Combine all the fillings together and melt in the microwave for 15–20 seconds until smooth. Use the rolling pin again to crush the biscuits in a heavy-duty freezer or sandwich bag.

6. In a large mixing bowl, place the cream cheese, granulated sweetener, powdered sweetener, vanilla extract and the melted Oreo filling and whisk until smooth. (Ensure the mixture is smooth with no lumps but be careful not to over whisk as you want to keep the mixture nice and thick.) Gently stir through the crushed biscuits.

7. Pour the cheesecake mixture onto the cooled cheesecake base, gently tap the tin on the work surface a few times to remove any big air bubbles and place in the fridge to set, ideally for 24 hours.

8. Once the cheesecake has set, remove it from the tin by carefully running a knife around the edge of the cheesecake before undoing the clasp on the side of the tin. Gently lift the tin away and very carefully slide the cheesecake onto a serving plate.

9. Melt the chocolate in the microwave for a few seconds (taking care not to burn it) and drizzle it over the top of the cheesecake using a teaspoon or small piping bag, then crumble the last Oreo biscuit on top.

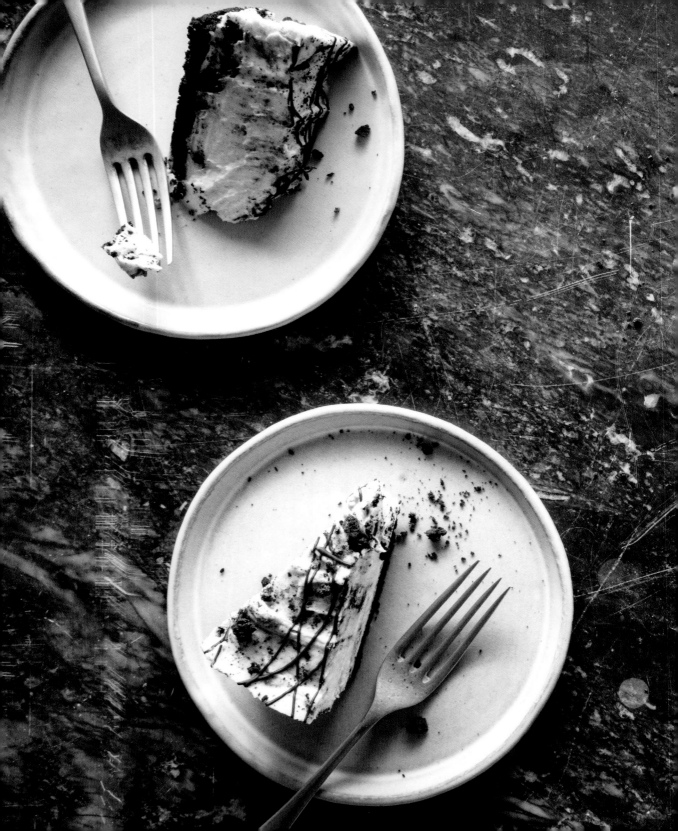

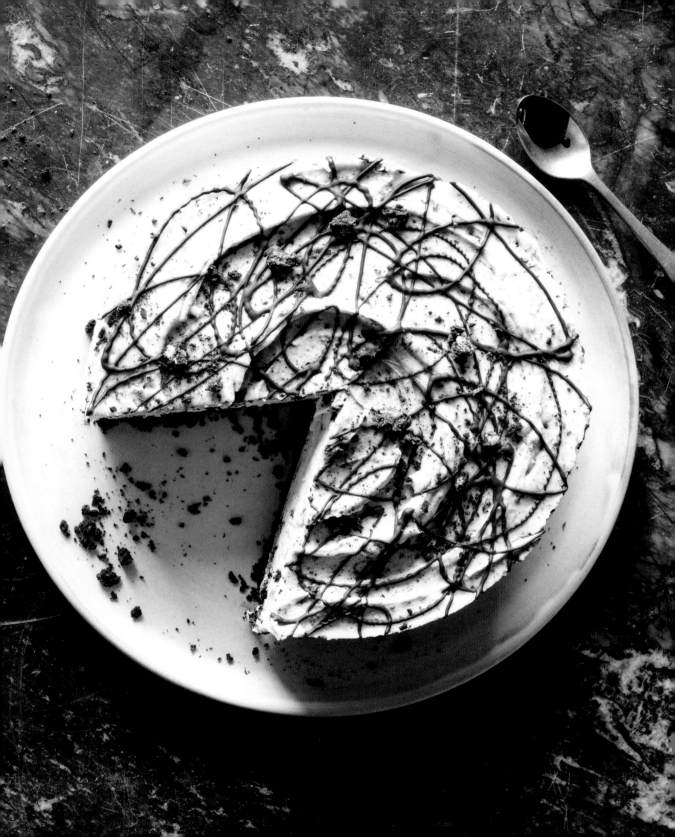

CALORIES 275
PROTEIN 8g
FAT 18g
CARBS 20g
SUGAR 10g

SERVES 12

PLANT-BASED JAMMY DODGER PROTEIN MINI CHEESECAKES

Preparation time: 20 minutes +
    3 hours soaking
Setting time: 3–4 hours

200g cashew nuts
100g frozen raspberries
250ml coconut cream
250ml plain dairy-free yogurt
1 tsp vanilla extract
2 Jammy Dodger biscuits
1 scoop (25g) vanilla protein
    powder
1 tbsp maple syrup
12 mini Jammy Dodger biscuits

FOR THE BASE
50g blanched almonds
2 tbsp maple syrup
6 Jammy Dodger biscuits

Jammy Dodgers are the ultimate British biscuit, with their sweet, vanilla, moreish flavour and memorable sticky raspberry jam filling! What's more, they are also vegan friendly and perfect for creating the most nostalgic mini cheesecakes that you can't help but smile when you make them!

1. Prepare the cashew nuts for the filling by leaving them to soak in a bowl of water for 3 hours.

2. To make the base, blitz together the almonds, maple syrup and 6 Jammy Dodgers in a food processor until fine tacky crumbs form.

3. Divide the base mixture between a 12-cavity mini cheesecake tin with removable bases and use your hands to press the biscuit base into each cavity.

4. Place the frozen raspberries in a saucepan and heat over a medium heat until the raspberries break down. Spoon a teaspoon of the raspberry mix into each cheesecake cavity, spreading it evenly over the base. Place the cheesecake tin in the freezer while you prepare the filling.

5. Drain the soaked cashew nuts and place in a food processor. Blitz together with the coconut cream, yogurt, vanilla extract, protein powder, 2 Jammy Dodgers and maple syrup until creamy and smooth.

6. Remove the mini cheesecake tin from the freezer and divide the filling between the 12 cavities then return the cheesecakes to the freezer for a further 3–4 hours. After 90 minutes place a mini Jammy Dodger on the top of each cheesecake then leave to finish freezing.

7. Once frozen, remove the cheesecakes from the freezer and let rest for 10–15 minutes or until they have thawed just enough to loosen easily from the mini tins. Pop out the cheesecakes and serve.

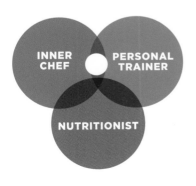

INNER CHEF

PERSONAL TRAINER

NUTRITIONIST

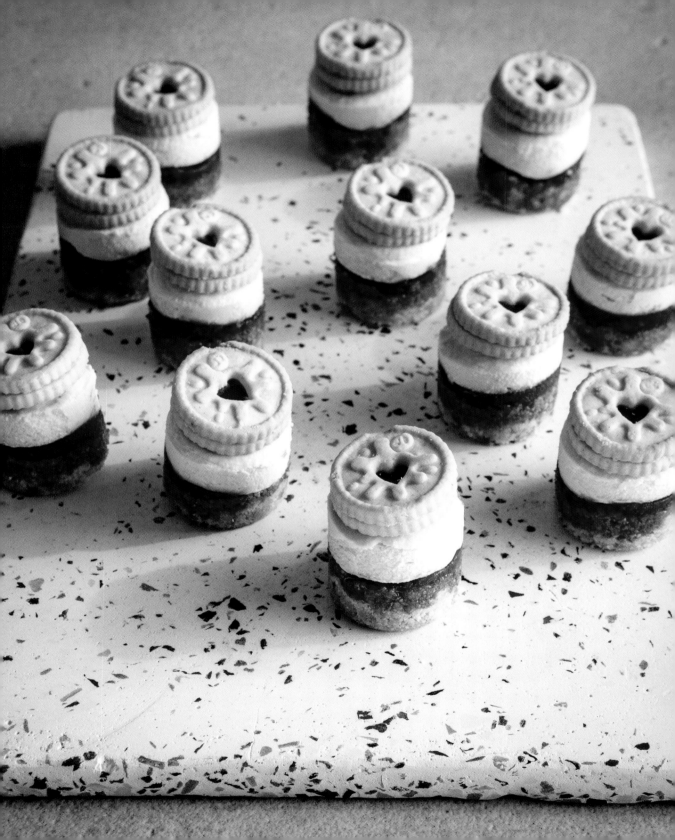

CALORIES 235
PROTEIN 11.2g
FAT 6.7g
CARBS 28.1g
SUGAR 6.7g

SERVES 10

Preparation time: 30 minutes
Cooking time: 20 minutes
Setting time: 24 hours

FOR THE OATY BANANA BASE
1 small ripe banana
200ml almond milk
200g jumbo rolled oats
1 tsp baking powder

FOR THE FILLING
4 gelatine sheets
1 small ripe banana
500g fat-free quark
400g light soft cheese
80g zero-calorie granulated
   white or brown sugar replacer
20g low-calorie caramel spread
   or syrup
100ml soya milk

FOR THE TOPPING
1 banana
25g low-calorie banoffee or
   caramel syrup
30g low-calorie caramel spread
   or syrup

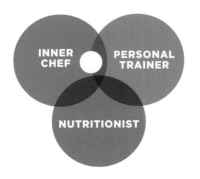

OATY BASE BANOFFEE CHEESECAKE

Naturally high in protein, the reason this is such a strong cheesecake is because, instead of the conventional biscuit base, the bottom of this culinary creation has been designed to more closely resemble a softer cakey structure. This makes it a smoother eat and it works brilliantly with the creamy toffee, caramel and banana flavours. Of course, if you guys want to switch a biscuit base back in, follow the No-bake Lemon & Blueberry Cheesecake biscuit base recipe on page 192.

1. Preheat the oven to 180°C/160°C fan/gas 4 and line a 23-cm round springform cake tin with parchment paper.

2. To make the base, mash the banana in a bowl and mix in the almond milk, rolled oats and baking powder. Pour the mixture into the lined tin and spread it out evenly. Place in the preheated oven and bake for 20 minutes until springy to touch. Remove from the oven and place the tin on a wire rack to cool completely.

3. Once the base has cooled, start preparing the filling. Place the gelatine sheets in a bowl of cold water and set aside to soak for 5 minutes to soften.

4. Mash the banana in a mixing bowl then add the remainder of the filling ingredients, apart from the milk, and whisk together until just fully combined. Be careful not to over mix as you do not want the mixture to become too liquid – you want to keep it as thick as possible.

5. Heat the milk in a small saucepan over a medium heat to just below boiling point, then take off the heat. Squeeze the excess cold water from the gelatine sheets and place in the hot milk, stirring the mixture for a few seconds until the gelatine dissolves.

6. Pour the milk with gelatine straight into the cheesecake mix and whisk together immediately (otherwise the gelatine will go stringy if cooled and left too long before mixing).

7. Pour the cheesecake mixture onto the cheesecake base, gently tap the tin on the work surface a few times to remove any big air bubbles and place in the fridge to set. It is best

to let the cheesecake set for at least 24 hours or even a little longer. (As this recipe contains low-fat alternatives, this cheesecake does tend to take longer to set than say a normal one with a very high fat content.)

8. Once the cheesecake has set, remove it from the tin by carefully running a knife around the edge of the cheesecake before undoing the clasp on the side of the tin. Gently lift the tin away and very carefully slide the cheesecake onto a serving plate.

9. To decorate, slice the banana into a small bowl, mix together with the banoffee or caramel syrup and spoon the syrupy bananas over the cheesecake. Melt the caramel spread in the microwave for a few seconds then drizzle over the top using a teaspoon or small piping bag. Place the cheesecake back in the fridge for half an hour before serving.

CALORIES 186
PROTEIN 13g
FAT 11g
CARBS 18g
SUGAR 14g

SERVES
8

Preparation time: 15 minutes
Cooking time: 50 minutes
Setting time: 3 hours

600g Philadelphia Lightest
cream cheese (or other
low-fat cream cheese), at
room temperature
180g zero-calorie granulated
white sugar replacer
2 tsp vanilla bean paste
3 eggs
300ml sour cream, at room
temperature
20g cornflour, sifted
2 scoops (50g) vanilla protein
powder
8 tsp Sweet Freedom low-
calorie caramel or popcorn
syrup, to serve
Vanilla Pod Ice Cream, to serve
(optional)

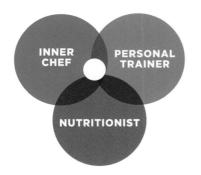

INNER
CHEF   PERSONAL
TRAINER

NUTRITIONIST

PROTEIN VANILLA POD BASQUE BURNT CHEESECAKE

In my opinion, the only way cheesecake could be made better is if you added custard and then enhanced it with protein. This is why I asked Hester to create a protein-enriched, Vanilla Pod Basque Burnt Cheesecake. This sweet, vanilla, melt-in-your-mouth, baked cheesecake is unbelievably low in calories for a slice, which could also be classed as your protein snack of the day. Top tip; if you can find a low-sugar popcorn syrup to drizzle over the top, you won't regret it!

1. Preheat the oven to 180°C/160°C fan/gas 4 and line a 20-cm round springform cake tin with a large piece of parchment paper, making sure it lines the whole of the tin, including the sides.

2. Use a hand-held electric mixer to whisk together the cream cheese, sweetener and vanilla bean paste in a large bowl then add the eggs, one by one, making sure each egg has been fully incorporated before adding the next.

3. Whisk in the sour cream then slow down the mixer speed and add the cornflour and protein powder and beat until fully blended.

4. Scrape down the bowl to ensure no ingredients are stuck at the bottom and mix everything together once more.

5. Pour the cheesecake mix into the lined tin and lightly tap the tin on a work surface to release any air bubbles. Place in the oven for 50 minutes.

6. When the cheesecake is baked the top will look a little burnt and it will be a little wobbly, but don't worry, it's meant to be like that! Place the tin on a cooling rack and leave to set and cool for at least 3 hours.

7. Once cooled, remove the cheesecake from the tin and place on a serving plate. This cheesecake works so well served with the Vanilla Pod Ice Cream (see page 188) or with a low-calorie caramel or popcorn syrup.

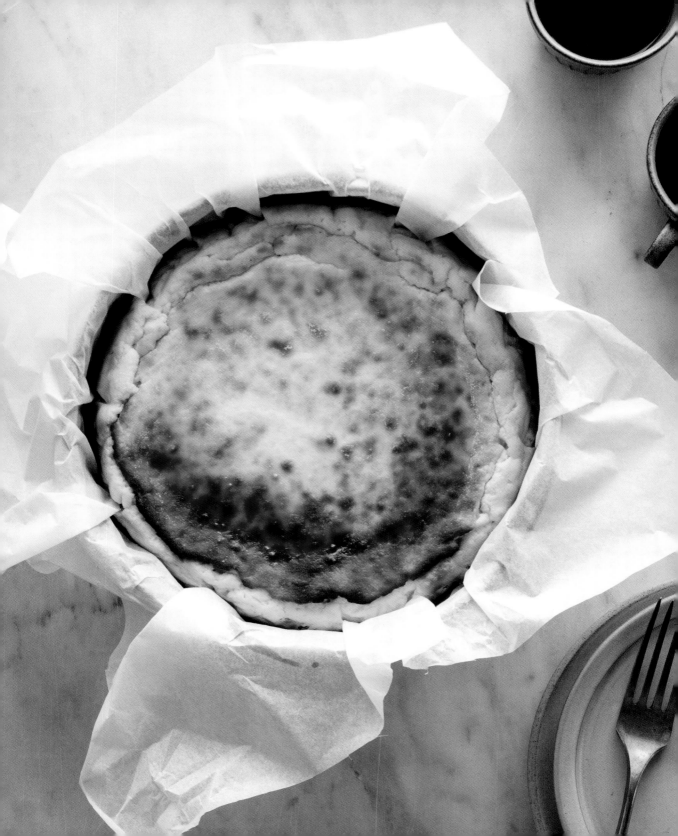

CALORIES 238
PROTEIN 13g
FAT 10g
CARBS 31g
SUGAR 14g

SERVES 10

NO-BAKE BISCOFF CHEESECAKE

Preparation time: 40 minutes
Setting time: 24 hours

FOR THE BISCUIT BASE
23 Lotus Biscoff biscuits
30g coconut oil

FOR THE FILLING
4 gelatine sheets
500g fat-free quark
400g Philadelphia Lightest
    cream cheese (or other
    low-fat cream cheese)
100g zero-calorie granulated
    white sugar replacer
45g Lotus Biscoff smooth spread
1 tsp vanilla extract
100ml soya milk

TO DECORATE
15g Lotus Biscoff smooth spread,
    to drizzle
2 Lotus Biscoff biscuits, crushed

I LOVE BISCOFF CARAMELISED BISCUITS. Created in 1932 in a Belgian bakery, traditionally they're flavoured with cinnamon, nutmeg, ginger and lots of other ingredients that your taste buds will love. But the only thing I like more than Biscoff biscuits ... is Biscoff cheesecake! High in protein, the caramelised biscuit base is layered with a soft, sweet, cream cheese Biscoff filling and, incredibly, our version only contains 238 calories per slice.

1. Place the biscuits in a heavy-duty freezer or sandwich bag and crush with a rolling pin until you have fine crumbs. Melt the coconut oil in the microwave in 7-second intervals until melted. Pour the crushed biscuits and the coconut oil into a bowl and mix together until the crumbs are fully coated in the oil.

2. Tip the crumbs into a lined 23-cm round springform cake tin, and use your hands to press the crumbs firmly and evenly into the base of the tin. Place in the fridge for 40 minutes to firm up.

3. To make the filling, place the gelatine sheets in a bowl of cold water and set aside to soak for 5 minutes to soften.

4. Place the quark, cream cheese, sweetener, Biscoff spread and vanilla extract into a large mixing bowl and whisk until fully combined. (Try to whisk for as little time as possible to ensure the mixture doesn't become too runny.)

5. Heat the milk in a small saucepan over a medium heat to just below boiling point then take off the heat. Squeeze the excess cold water from the gelatine sheets and place in the hot milk, stirring the mixture for a few seconds until the gelatine dissolves.

6. Pour the milk with gelatine straight into the cheesecake mix and whisk together immediately (otherwise the gelatine will go stringy if cooled and left too long before mixing).

7. Pour the cheesecake mixture onto the chilled biscuit base, gently tap the tin on the work surface a few times to remove any big air bubbles and place in the fridge to set for at least 24 hours. (These cheesecakes take a little longer to set than normal because of the low percentage of fat and sugar in the recipe. Fat and sugar are usually used not just for flavour but also to help hold the structure of the cheesecake.)

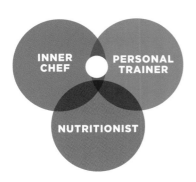

INNER CHEF
PERSONAL TRAINER
NUTRITIONIST

8. Once the cheesecake is set, remove it from the tin by carefully running a knife around the edge of the cheesecake before undoing the clasp on the side of the tin. Gently lift the tin away and very carefully slide the cheesecake onto a serving plate.

9. Melt the Biscoff spread in the microwave for a few seconds and, either with a teaspoon or small piping bag, drizzle the sauce over the top then sprinkle over the crushed biscuits to finish.

Protein Snacks

This part of the book can only be described as gourmet sports snacks at their very best. Backed by nutritional science, it takes the principle of a conventional protein snack and completely reinvents it with protein cookie dough, brookies and pronuts. Essentially, your kitchen cupboard and gym bag will never be the same again.

CALORIES 91
PROTEIN 16g
FAT 1g
CARBS 5g
SUGARS 3g

SERVES 4

Preparation time: 10 minutes
Setting time: overnight/8 hours

3 scoops (75g) strawberry
   protein powder
12g sachet gelatine powder
100ml hot water
25g fresh blueberries
30g fresh raspberries
4 strawberries, quartered

ANGEL DELIGHT PROTEIN JELLY

Most people have enjoyed a bowl of Angel Delight in their time – whether you're a child or an adult – and some of us are guilty of eating the whole packet by ourselves! Well, this recipe is all about nostalgia … recreating this memorable pudding for a fraction of the calories, but with a lot more protein. Basically, if you're wanting to eat clean, but need to have that sweet fix, then look no further.

1. Whisk 450ml of cold water and the strawberry protein powder together in a mixing bowl then add the gelatine powder and stir with a balloon whisk to combine.

2. Use a jelly mould of your choice or individual serving glasses and place a good handful of the fresh fruit into each of the moulds then pour in the strawberry jelly mixture.

3. Place in the fridge for at least 8 hours to set, preferably overnight, before serving.

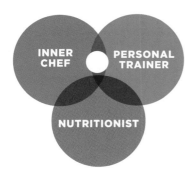

INNER CHEF

PERSONAL TRAINER

NUTRITIONIST

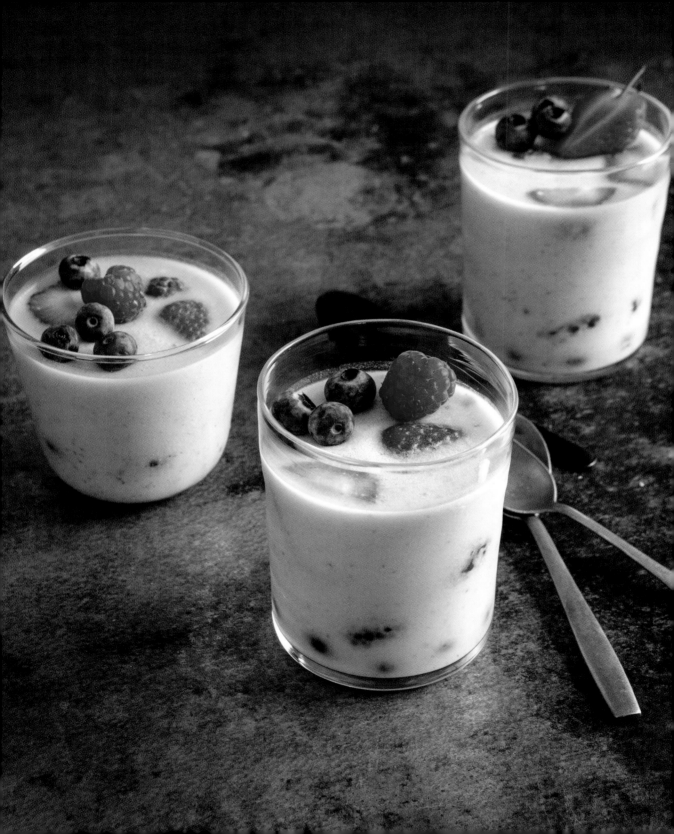

**SERVES
9**

JAMMY BAKEWELL PROTEIN SQUARES

Preparation time: 10 minutes
Cooking time: 20 minutes

80g rolled oats
6 scoops (150g) cherry bakewell or vanilla protein powder
40g zero-calorie granulated brown sugar replacer
40g zero-calorie granulated white sugar replacer
50g pecans, chopped
120g Flora light spread (or other light spread)
200g reduced-sugar raspberry jam

Jammy Bakewell Protein Squares were inspired by a childhood favourite of ours called a jam roly-poly. Tasting like pure nostalgia, this traditional British pudding was invented in the 19th century and had remained relatively unchanged for many years. But we decided to take the recipe, reverse engineer it and add a generous serving of quality protein, all so you can eat like an elite athlete and a kid at the same time.

1. Preheat the oven to 180°C/160°C fan/gas 4.

2. In a large mixing bowl, mix together the oats, protein powder, sweeteners and chopped pecans. Use your hands to rub the mixture together with the spread until it has a rough crumb texture.

3. Place three-quarters of the mixture into a lined 20 x 20-cm square baking tin and use your hands to firmly press it into the base of the tin.

4. Spread the raspberry jam over the base then scatter the remaining crumble evenly over the top.

5. Place in the oven for 20 minutes until the top has turned golden brown.

6. Remove from the oven and leave to cool until just warm then cut into nine squares. Serve as a pudding with custard, if you like, or eat as a snack just as it is.

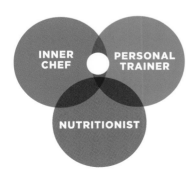

INNER CHEF
PERSONAL TRAINER
NUTRITIONIST

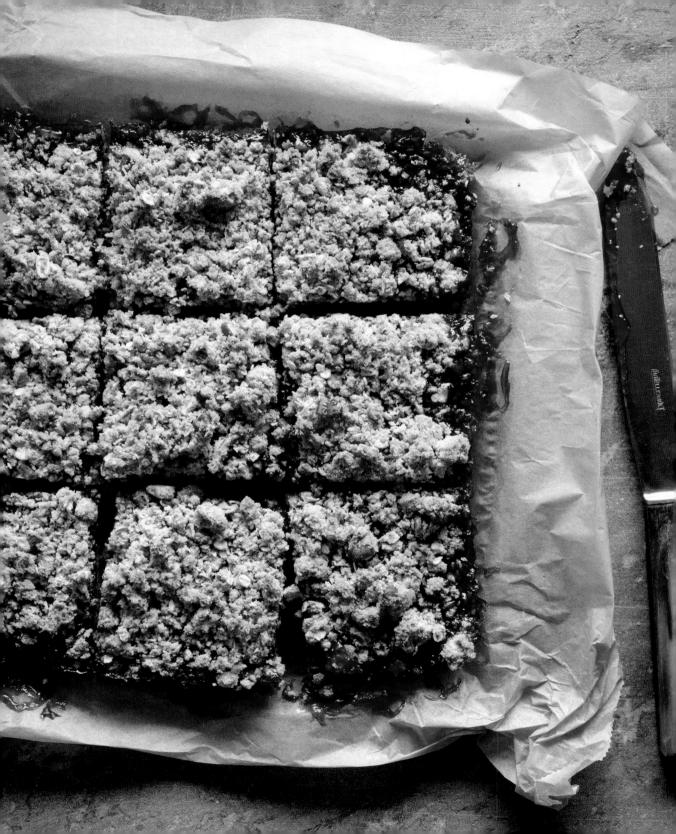

CALORIES 218
PROTEIN 13g
FAT 13g
CARBS 12g
SUGARS 11g

SERVES
9

COOKIE DOUGH PROTEIN BARS

Preparation time: 15 minutes
Freezing time: 40 minutes

50g light agave syrup
150g almond butter
1 tsp vanilla extract
4 scoops (100g) vanilla protein
   powder
80ml soya milk
1 tsp cookie dough flavouring
   (optional)
30g milk chocolate chips
50g dark chocolate

This might be one of the best-tasting ways to ensure you hit your elevated protein requirements for the day. They are really easy to make (and can be stored in the fridge for throughout the week) and they are also quite calorific, so are best eaten during those periods of high-volume training when you need both the calories and protein to help you recover.

1. Line a 20 x 20-cm square baking tin with parchment paper and set aside.

2. In a small bowl, mix together the agave syrup, almond butter, vanilla extract, protein powder, soya milk and cookie dough flavouring, if using. Finally, mix in the milk chocolate chips. The mixture should look like a cookie dough.

3. Place the mixture in the lined baking tin and use your hands to press the dough into the tin. It should be quite a thin layer of cookie dough (about 1cm thick).

4. Place the dark chocolate in a heatproof bowl over a pan of simmering water, making sure it doesn't touch the water. Gently melt the chocolate, stirring occasionally. (Alternatively, place the bowl in a microwave and heat for no more than 6 seconds at a time, stirring each time until the chocolate has fully melted, taking care not to burn it.) Pour the melted dark chocolate over the cookie dough and carefully spread it out evenly over the top.

5. Place in the freezer for about 40 minutes, until the cookie is firm enough to slice, then cut into nine squares for a fulfilling snack on-the-go. If you want to reduce calories, cut into 12 servings instead for a healthy treat-sized snack.

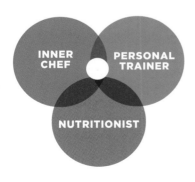

INNER CHEF
PERSONAL TRAINER
NUTRITIONIST

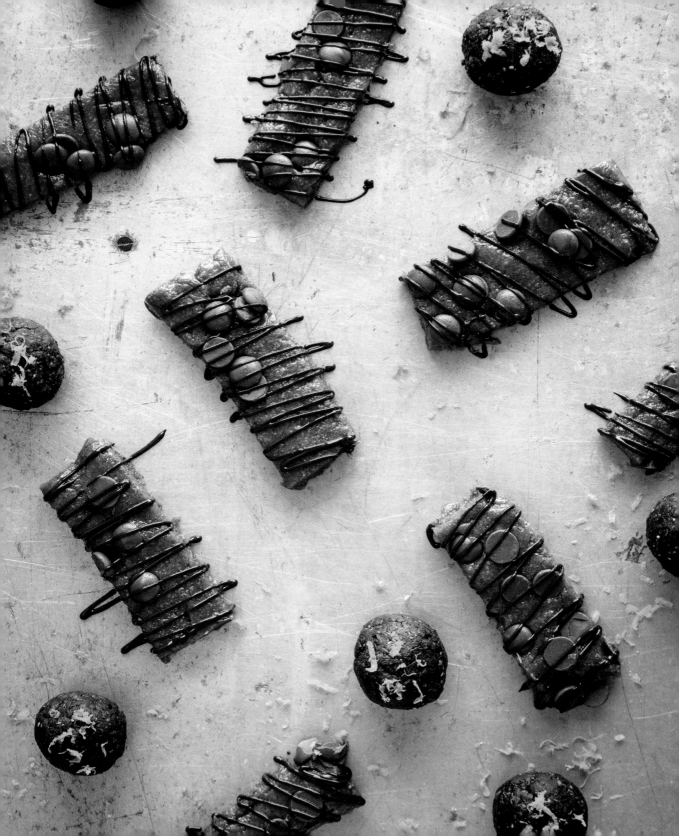

CALORIES 153
PROTEIN 2g
FAT 7g
CARBS 20g
SUGARS 16g

SERVES
18

Preparation time: 30 mins + chilling

100g Terry's Chocolate Orange
50ml maple syrup
100g medjool dates, pitted
100g raisins
25g cocoa powder
20g coconut oil, melted
30g cashew butter
25g super greens powder
50g Ready Brek (or other instant oats)
20g ground flaxseeds
20g chia seeds

TO DECORATE
100g dark chocolate, broken into small pieces
zest of 1 orange

CHOCOLATE ORANGE ENERGY BALLS

This recipe packs so many calories, carbs and micronutrients into every single serving and is ideal when you're stepping up the volume and intensity of your endurance training. Whether running a marathon or competing in a triathlon, these Chocolate Orange Energy Balls taste incredible and are a great natural alternative to many synthetic energy gels. See photo on previous page.

1. Place the Terry's Chocolate Orange in a heatproof bowl over a pan of simmering water, making sure it doesn't touch the water. Gently melt the chocolate, stirring occasionally. (Alternatively, place the bowl in a microwave and heat for no more than 6 seconds at a time, stirring each time until the chocolate has fully melted, taking care not to burn it.)

2. Place the melted chocolate in a food processor, along with the remainder of the ingredients and pulse until the mixture is uniform and well combined.

3. Roll the mixture into 18 balls (each about the size of a Brussels sprout) and place onto a baking sheet lined with parchment paper. Place in the freezer for an hour (this helps them keep their shape when coating them in chocolate).

4. Melt the dark chocolate in a bowl and use a teaspoon to help you roll each ball around in the melted chocolate until it is completely coated. Place the balls back onto the lined baking sheet and sprinkle with a little orange zest (this bit is optional and mainly decorative, but does make them look awesome!).

5. Leave the chocolate energy balls in the fridge to set for 1–2 hours and enjoy!

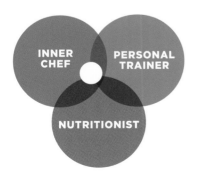

INNER CHEF

PERSONAL TRAINER

NUTRITIONIST

CALORIES 280
PROTEIN 22g
FAT 12g
CARBS 19g
SUGARS 17g

SERVES
4

TRIPLE CHOCOLATE PROTEIN MOUSSE

Preparation time: 15 minutes +
overnight chilling

50g white chocolate
550ml soya milk
3 scoops (75g) vanilla protein
powder
1 tsp vanilla bean paste
12g sachet gelatine powder

TO DECORATE
25g milk chocolate, melted
25g dark chocolate, melted
12g chocolate crispies or
other chocolate decorations
(optional)

This light and fluffy white-chocolate mousse is topped with melted milk and dark chocolate and is one of the most indulgent ways to get 22g of protein (per serving) into your diet. We usually have this as a dessert, but it can also be eaten throughout the day if you need to curb your cravings with a healthy, sweet, protein-packed snack.

1. Place the chocolate in a heatproof bowl over a pan of simmering water, making sure it doesn't touch the water. Gently melt the chocolate, stirring occasionally. (Alternatively, place the bowl in a microwave and heat for no more than 6 seconds at a time, stirring each time until the chocolate has fully melted, taking care not to burn it.)

2. In a large jug, mix together the soya milk, protein powder, melted white chocolate and vanilla bean paste.

3. Pour 100ml of boiling water in a small bowl and add the gelatine powder. Stir until the gelatine has completely dissolved then pour into the mousse mixture and stir until fully combined.

4. Pour the mousse mixture into four pudding pots and place in the fridge to set overnight.

5. Remove from the fridge and drizzle the melted chocolate over the top to decorate. Finish with some extra chocolate decorations of your choice, if you fancy!

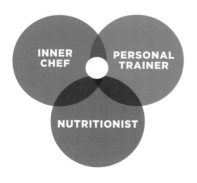

INNER CHEF

PERSONAL TRAINER

NUTRITIONIST

CALORIES 103
PROTEIN 8g
FAT 4g
CARBS 14g
SUGARS 3g

SERVES 12

PRONUTS

Preparation time: 20 minutes
Cooking time: 10–15 minutes

100ml liquid egg whites
100g oat flour (oats blitzed in a food processor)
150g apple sauce
4 scoops (100g) vanilla protein powder
1 tsp bicarbonate of soda

FOR THE GLAZE
30g coconut oil
50g zero-calorie granulated brown sugar replacer
1 tsp ground cinnamon

We're so proud of our Pronuts! This is because usually adding protein powder to a recipe can make it dense, chewy and heavy on the stomach – but not these. Light, fluffy and packing 8g of protein into every serving, your taste buds will barely recognise these from the sugar-filled, full-fat originals. Top tip: be sure to use a silicone doughnut mould rather than a tin, as your batter will bake too quickly and become hard.

1. Preheat the oven to 180°C/160°C fan/gas 4.

2. Using a hand-held electric mixer, whisk the egg whites in a clean mixing bowl until they become glossy and stiff peaks form, then set aside.

3. In a separate bowl, mix together the oat flour, apple sauce, protein powder and bicarbonate of soda.

4. Use a silicone spatula to gently fold in the whipped egg whites, taking care not to knock the air bubbles out of the mixture. This is what is going to make the doughnuts nice and light.

5. Pour the mixture into 12 silicone ring-doughnut moulds and place in the oven for 10–15 minutes, until risen and golden. Remove from the oven and leave to cool in the moulds until cool enough to handle.

6. The top side of the doughnuts will have risen and won't look like a ring doughnut, however, when the doughnuts are turned out of the tin the ring shape created by the mould can be seen. This is the top side of the doughnut, ready for glazing and decorating.

7. In a small bowl, melt the coconut oil for a few seconds in the microwave. In a separate shallow bowl or plate, mix together the sweetener and cinnamon.

8. Quickly dip the top side of each doughnut in the melted coconut oil, lightly coating the surface, then immediately dip in the sweetener and cinnamon mix to coat. Enjoy while still warm and the aroma of cinnamon fills the kitchen.

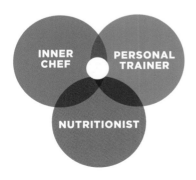

INNER CHEF

PERSONAL TRAINER

NUTRITIONIST

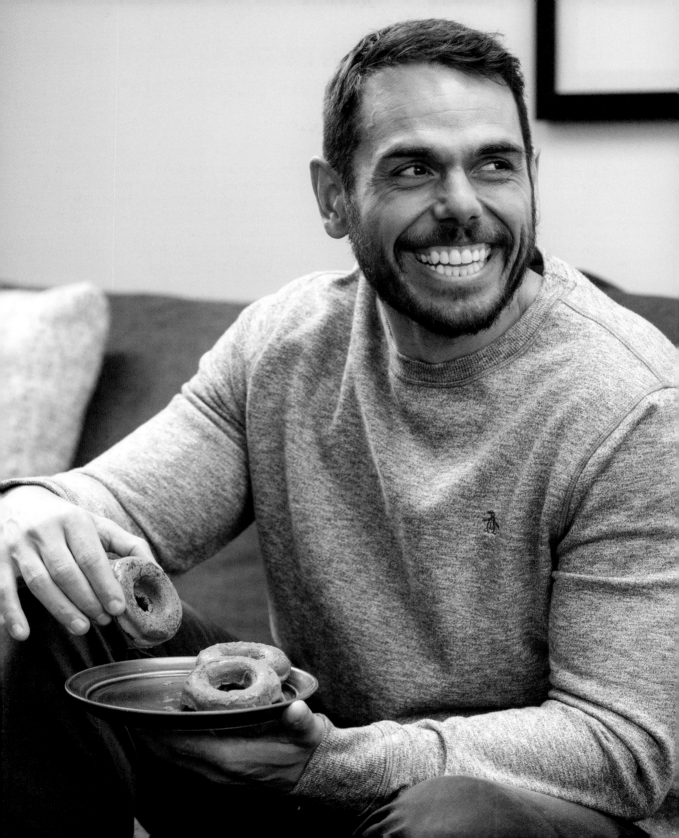

CALORIES 364
PROTEIN 35g
FAT 13g
CARBS 15g
SUGARS 13g

SERVES
2

STRAWBERRY PRO-FRAPPUCCINO

Preparation time: 5 minutes

¼ tub (250g) Vanilla Pod Ice Cream (see page 188)
450ml almond milk
100g strawberries, stalks removed
200g ice cubes
2 scoops (50g) strawberry protein powder
200ml Elmlea single light cream 45% less fat
a few strawberries, to decorate

If there was a race for the quickest time to prepare a protein-packed breakfast, this would win. Made with fresh strawberries, so it's naturally loaded with antioxidants, it's perfect if you're in a rush and need 35g of quality protein as quickly and efficiently as possible.

1. Place all the ingredients in a blender and blitz for a minute or so until smooth and creamy. Pour into a glass and top with a few extra strawberries.

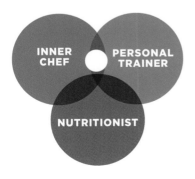

INNER CHEF
PERSONAL TRAINER
NUTRITIONIST

COCONUT & RASPBERRY PROTEIN LOAF CAKE

SERVES 10

Preparation time: 10 minutes +
1 hour resting
Cooking time: 45–50 minutes

250ml coconut plant-milk
alternative
150g tinned coconut milk
80ml agave syrup
60g desiccated coconut
40g zero-calorie granulated
white sugar replacer
250g self-raising flour
1 tsp baking powder
2 scoops (50g) vanilla protein
powder

TO DECORATE
50g raspberry jam
10g desiccated coconut

You'll often find more of these protein loaf cakes in our house than loaves of bread. This is because the coconut and raspberry complement each other perfectly, especially when the recipe is cooked to a golden-brown texture and served piping hot straight out of the oven. But, also, because this can be easily prepared at the weekend, divided into portions and eaten throughout the week to ensure you're hitting your protein requirements for the day.

1. In a bowl, whisk together both the coconut milks, agave syrup and desiccated coconut. Leave to rest for 1 hour to allow the desiccated coconut to soften and release more of its flavour.

2. Preheat the oven to 170°C/150°C fan/gas 3 and line a 900g loaf cake tin.

3. Mix together the sweetener, self-raising flour, baking powder and protein powder in a large mixing bowl. Pour in the coconut mixture and stir everything together until a smooth cake batter forms.

4. Pour the coconut cake batter into the lined loaf tin and bake in the oven for 45–50 minutes until a skewer inserted into the centre of the cake comes out clean. If the top of the cake is browning too quickly, gently place a piece of aluminium foil over the top to stop it colouring any more.

5. Remove from the oven and leave the loaf to cool in its tin for a few hours. When cool, place on a serving plate and poke 6 holes into the loaf cake with a skewer. Fill a piping bag with 30g of raspberry jam, and pipe the jam into the holes. Spread the remaining jam all over the top of the cake before sprinkling over the desiccated coconut.

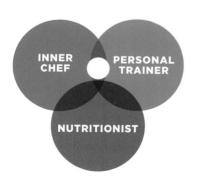

INNER CHEF

PERSONAL TRAINER

NUTRITIONIST

CALORIES 286
PROTEIN 11g
FAT 17g
CARBS 23g
SUGARS 15g

SERVES
8

MALTESER PROTEIN BLONDIE CUPS

Preparation time: 10 minutes
Cooking time: 12–15 minutes

75g maple syrup
130g cashew butter
50g ground almonds
30g Horlicks Light powder
200ml oat milk
2 scoops (45g) vanilla protein powder
50g Maltesers, crushed
30g milk chocolate

Quite possibly the greatest snack ever to be served in a mug, these Malteser Protein Blondie Cups taste incredible when served straight out of the oven. Packing a massive 11g of quality protein in just one serving, they've become our favourite snack to eat following a cold ice swim or frosty trail run.

1. Preheat the oven to 180°C/160°C fan/gas 4 and line eight cavities of a muffin tin with paper cases.

2. Place the maple syrup, cashew butter, ground almonds, Horlicks powder, oat milk and protein powder in a mixing bowl and use a hand-held electric mixer to whisk together to form a gooey brownie mix.

3. Mix in the crushed Maltesers and divide the mixture evenly between the eight paper cases, then place in the oven for 12–15 minutes.

4. At the end of the cooking time the blondie should be crispy on top but still a little gooey and soft in the middle. Remove the blondies from the oven and allow to cool a little.

5. While the blondies are cooling, place the chocolate in a heatproof bowl over a pan of simmering water, making sure it doesn't touch the water. Gently melt the chocolate, stirring occasionally. (Alternatively, place the bowl in a microwave and heat for no more than 6 seconds at a time, stirring each time until the chocolate has fully melted, taking care not to burn it.) Drizzle the melted milk chocolate over the top of the blondies for extra chocolatelyness!

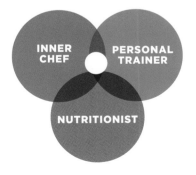

INNER CHEF

PERSONAL TRAINER

NUTRITIONIST

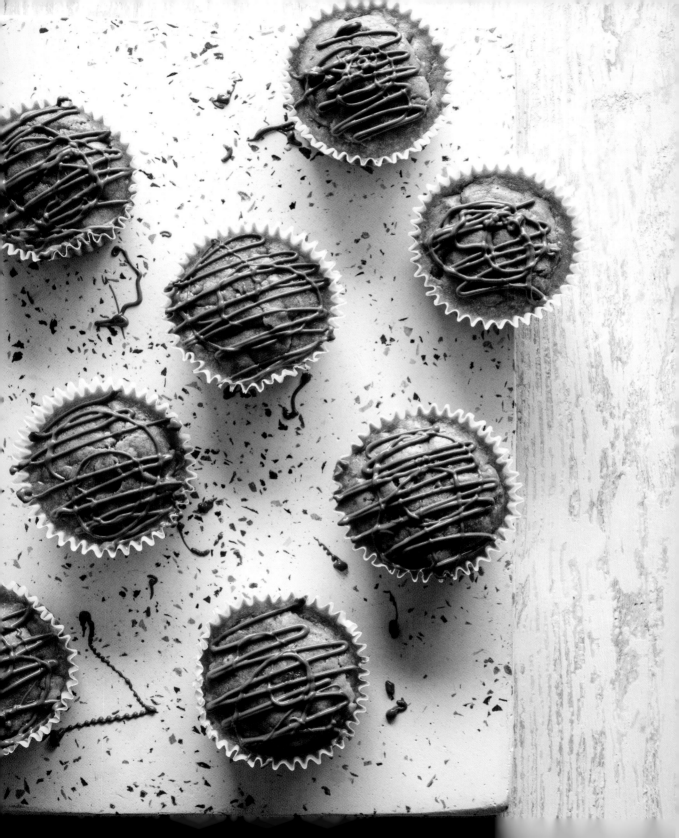

SERVES 9

PROTEIN BROOKIES

Preparation time: 15 minutes
Cooking time: 20–25 minutes

FOR THE COOKIE BASE
50g light agave syrup
150g almond butter
1 tsp vanilla extract
4 scoops (100g) vanilla protein powder
80ml soya milk
30g milk chocolate chips

FOR THE BROWNIE TOPPING
90g chocolate protein brownie mix
50g self-raising flour

TO DECORATE
30g dark chocolate chips

I love cookies and I love brownies. Which is why it only made logical sense to combine the two into a healthy, hybrid snack capable of supporting my elevated protein requirements for the day. Consisting of a soft, chewy cookie with a moist, chocolatey brownie top, it's then sprinkled with dark chocolate chips and contains an impressive 19g of protein per brookie. Honestly, these will revolutionise the contents of your cookie jar.

1. Preheat the oven to 180°C/160°C fan/gas 4 and line a 20 x 20-cm square baking tin with parchment paper.

2. In a mixing bowl, stir together the agave syrup, almond butter, vanilla extract, vanilla protein powder and soya milk. The mixture will come together to form a cookie dough paste. Finally, mix in the chocolate chips.

3. Place the cookie dough in the lined baking tin and press it into the base with your hands. It should be quite a thin layer of cookie dough (about 1cm thick).

4. For the topping, whisk the brownie mix and flour together with 150ml of water to make a smooth, thick batter then pour on top of the cookie dough, spreading it out evenly.

5. Finally, sprinkle the dark chocolate chips onto the surface of the brownie batter and place in the oven for 20–25 minutes, until the brownie batter is evenly baked.

6. Remove from the oven and allow to cool until just luke warm. Protein brownies bake a little differently to standard brownies and this will ensure the brookie has set before serving.

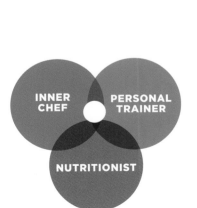

INNER CHEF

PERSONAL TRAINER

NUTRITIONIST

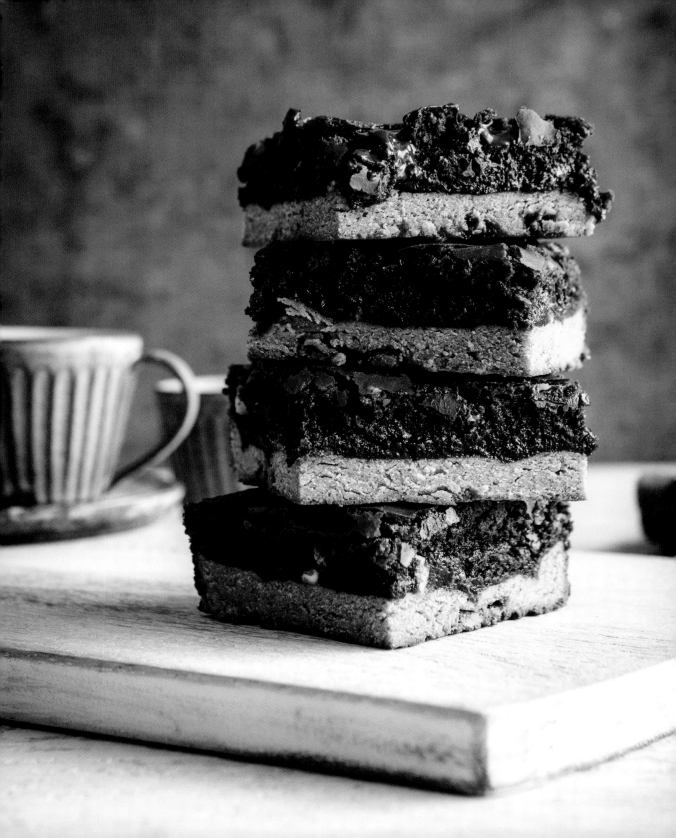

ENDNOTES

1   'Worldwide obesity has doubled since 1980.' The World Health Organization (February 2014)

2   Pozza C., Isidori A.M. 'What's behind the obesity epidemic.' (2018)

3   Traci Mann et al. 'Medicare's search for effective obesity treatments; diets are not the answer.' University of California, Los Angeles (2007)

4   Albert Stunkard, M.D and Mavis McClaren-Hume, M.S. 'The results of treatments for obesity: a review of the literature and report of a series.' (1959). Archives of Internal Medicine, 103(1):79–85. Although this report was published back in 1959 and based on a study with 100 patients, it's been reinforced by numerous clinical studies since 1959 and was recognised at the Australian New Zealand Obesity Society conference 2009 and the International Obesity Summit 2010.

5   Pankevich DE., Teegarden SL., Hedin AD., Jensen CL. and Bale TL. 'Caloric restriction experience reprograms stress and orexigenic pathways and promotes binge eating.' *The Journal of Neuroscience*, 2010 Dec 1;30(48):16399–407

6   Traci Mann et al. 'Medicare's search for effective obesity treatments; diets are not the answer.' University of California, Los Angeles (2007)

7   Stewart TM., Williamson DA. and White MA. 'Rigid vs. flexible dieting: association with eating disorder symptoms in non-obese women.' Appetite, 2002 Feb;38(1):39–44.

8   Alhassan S., Kim S., Bersamin A., King AC. and Gardner CD. 'Dietary adherence and weight loss success among overweight women: results from the A TO Z weight loss study.' *International Journal of Obesity* (2008) 32, 985–991

9   Beecher GR., Stewart KK., Holden JM., Harnly JM. and Wolf WR. 'Legacy of Wilbur O. Atwater: human nutrition research expansion at the USDA--interagency development of food composition research.' The Journal of Nutrition, 2009 Jan;139(1):178-84.

10 Schoeller D A. 'The energy balance equation: looking back and looking forward are two very different views.' *Nutrition Reviews*, 2009 May;67(5):249–54

11 Burke LM, Cox GR, Culmmings NK and Desbrow B. 'Guidelines for daily carbohydrate intake: do athletes achieve them?' *Sports Medicine*, 2001;31(4):267–99.

12 Schoeller DA. and Buchholz AC. 'Energetics of obesity and weight control: does diet composition matter?' *The Journal of the American Dietetic Association*, 2005 May;105(5 Suppl 1):S24–8.

13 Lambert EV, Speechly DP, Dennis SC, and Noakes TD. 'Enhanced endurance in trained cyclists during moderate intensity exercise following 2 weeks adaptation to a high fat diet.' *European Journal of Applied Physiology and Occupational Physiology,* October 1994, Volume 69, Issue 4, pp287–293

14 Kaidar-Person O., Person B., Szomstein S. and Rosenthal RJ. 'Nutritional deficiencies in morbidly obese patients: a new form of malnutrition? Part A: vitamins.' Obesity Surgery, 2008 Jul;18(7):870–6.

15 Kaidar-Person O. and Rosenthal RJ. 'Malnutrition in morbidly obese patients: fact or fiction?' *Minerva Chirurgica*, 2009 Jun; 64(3):297–302.

16 Balsom PD, Gaitanos GC, Söderlund K, Ekblom B. 'High-intensity exercise and muscle glycogen availability in humans.' *Acta Physioligca Scandinavia*, 1999 Apr;165(4):337–45.

17 Burke LM, Cox GR, Culmmings NK and Desbrow B. 'Guidelines for daily carbohydrate intake: do athletes achieve them?' *Sports Medicine*, 2001;31(4):267–99.

18 Estelle V. Lambert, David P. Speechly, Steven C. Dennis, Timothy and D. Noakes. 'Enhanced endurance in trained cyclists during moderate intensity exercise following 2 weeks adaptation to a high fat diet.' *European Journal of Applied Physiology and Occupational Physiology* October 1994, Volume 69, Issue 4, pp287–293.

19 R.C Brown. 'Nutrition for optimal performance during exercise: carbohydrate and fat.' *Current Sports Medicine Reports*, 2002 Aug;1(4):222–9.

CONVERSION CHARTS

DRY WEIGHTS

GRAMS (G)	OUNCES (OZ)
5	¼
8 / 10	⅓
15	½
20	¾
25	1
30 / 35	1¼
40	1½
50	2
60 / 70	2½
75 / 85 / 90	3
100	3½
110 / 120	4
125 / 130	4½
135 / 140 / 150	5
170 / 175	6
200	7
225	8
250	9
265	9½
275	10
300	11
325	11½
350	12
375	13
400	14
425	15
450	1lb
475	1lb 1oz
500	1lb 2oz

GRAMS (G)	OUNCES (OZ)
550	1lb 3oz
600	1lb 5oz
625	1lb 6oz
650	1lb 7oz
675	1½lb
700	1lb 9oz
750	1lb 10oz
800	1¾lb
850	1lb 14oz
900	2lb
950	2lb 2oz
1kg	2lb 3oz
1.1kg	2lb 6oz
1.25kg	2¾lb
1.3 / 1.4kg	3lb
1.5kg	3lb 5oz
1.75 / 1.8kg	4lb
2kg	4lb 4oz
2.25kg	5lb
2.5kg	5½lb
3kg	6½lb
3.5kg	7¾lb
4kg	8¾lb
4.5kg	9¾lb
6.8kg	15lb
9kg	20lb

LIQUID MEASURES

568ml = 1 UK pint (20fl oz)

16fl oz = 1 US pint

METRIC (ML)	IMPERIAL (FL OZ)	CUPS
15	½	1 tbsp (level)
20	¾	
25	1	$^1/_8$
30	1¼	
50	2	¼
60	2½	
753		
100	3½	$^3/_8$
110 / 120	4	½
125	4½	
150	5	$^2/_3$
175	6	¾
200 / 215	7	
225	8	1
250	9	
275	9½	
300	½ pint	1¼
350	12	1½
375	13	
400	14	
425	15	
450	16	2
500	18	2¼
550	19	
600	1 pint	2½
700	1¼ pints	
750	1$^1/_3$ pints	
800	1 pint 9fl oz	
850	1½ pints	

METRIC (ML)	IMPERIAL (FL OZ)	CUPS
900	1 pint 12fl oz	3¾
1 litre	1¾ pints	1 quart (4 cups)
1.2 litres	2 pints	1¼ quarts
1.25 litres	2¼ pints	
1.5 litres	2½ pints	3 US pints
1.75 / 1.8 litres	3 pints	
2 litres	3½ pints	2 quarts
2.2 litres	3¾ pints	
2.5 litres	4 $^1/_3$ pints	
3 litres	5 pints	
3.5 litres	6 pints	

OVEN TEMPERATURES

°C	°F	GAS MARK	DESCRIPTION
110	225	¼	cool
130	250	½	cool
140	275	1	very low
150	300	2	very low
160 / 170	325	3	low to moderate
180	350	4	moderate
190	375	5	moderately hot
200	400	6	hot
220	425	7	hot
230	450	8	hot
240	475	9	very hot

INDEX

ACKNOWLEDGEMENTS

For as long as I can remember, my life has been entirely centred around food. Whether eating to fuel an ultra-marathon swim across oceans or attending a giant family feast to celebrate a birthday, I basically have a deep-rooted enthusiasm for everything that is edible. Why? Well, there are a few reasons, but the first is called Jacqueline Edgley ... also known as Mum. This is because the culinary creations that have emerged out of her kitchen over the years can only be described as legendary. Her Sunday roast dinners more closely resemble a king's banquet, her cheesecakes should be served with Michelin Stars and her homemade rice puddings smell like comfort and taste like a hug. In short, my mum's kitchen is one of my all-time favourite places to visit. It doesn't matter where I am in the world (from the Amazon rainforest to the Arctic circle) like a homing pigeon I will find my way home if I know a freshly baked pudding is coming out of the oven.

But simply having a love of food in all its forms isn't enough to publish a cookbook. No, see the primary (powerful) reason this came into existence is because of Hester Sabery ... also known as my girlfriend. She's basically a demigoddess of gastronomy who can take any unhealthy recipe, reverse engineer it and then reconstruct it into a healthy, nutrient-dense alternative. Put simply, she is the reason this book exists, since the recipes contained within these pages began as a set of scribbles on a notepad we keep in the kitchen cupboard, but thanks to her genius it evolved into something so much more.

Finally, I want to thank the amazing publishing team at HarperCollins who shared my vision to create a cookbook that would educate and empower millions and be the logical sequel to the *Sunday Times* bestseller, *The World's Fittest Book*. Although this was such an ambitious book to write, edit, format and photograph, I will be forever grateful to the time, resources and expertise they committed to making this a timeless literary tool for those who love food as much as they love fitness.

HarperCollins*Publishers*
1 London Bridge Street
London SE1 9GF

www.harpercollins.co.uk

HarperCollins*Publishers*
1st Floor, Watermarque Building, Ringsend Road
Dublin 4, Ireland

First published by HarperCollins*Publishers* 2022

10 9 8 7 6 5 4 3 2 1

Text © Ross Edgley 2022
Photography © Andrew Hayes-Watkins 2022
Except pages 15, 29 © James Appleton; pages 14, 22, 27, 30 © Simon Howard

Ross Edgley asserts the moral right to be identified as the author of this work

A catalogue record of this book is available from the British Library

ISBN 978-0-00-846561-2

Layout: Bobby Birchall, Bobby&Co
Food Stylist: Ellie Mulligan
Prop Stylist: Rachel Vere

Printed and bound by GPS Group

MIX
Paper from
responsible sources
FSC™ C007454

This book is produced from independently certified FSC™ paper to ensure responsible forest management.

For more information visit: www.harpercollins.co.uk/green

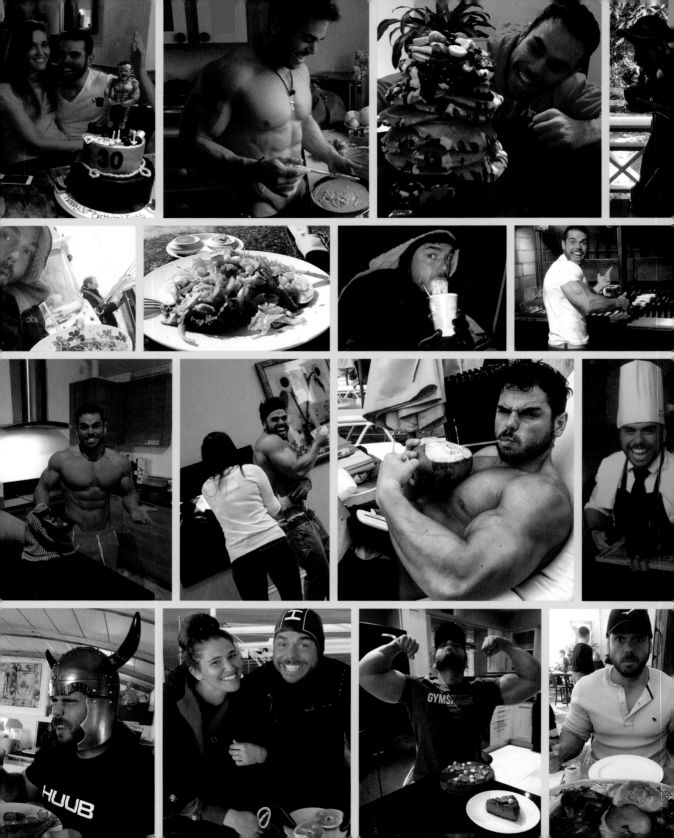